Safe Water, Sanitation, and Early Childhood Malnutrition in East Africa

Safe Water, Sanitation, and Early Childhood Malnutrition in East Africa

An African Feminist Analysis of the Lives of Women in Kenya, Tanzania, and Uganda

Edited by
Assata Zerai and Brenda N. Sanya

LEXINGTON BOOKS
Lanham • Boulder • New York • London

Published by Lexington Books
An imprint of The Rowman & Littlefield Publishing Group, Inc.
4501 Forbes Boulevard, Suite 200, Lanham, Maryland 20706
www.rowman.com

Unit A, Whitacre Mews, 26-34 Stannary Street, London SE11 4AB

British Library Cataloguing in Publication Information Available

Library of Congress Cataloging-in-Publication Data

ISBN: 978-1-4985-2083-6 (cloth : alk. paper)
ISBN: 978-1-4985-2084-3 (electronic)

∞™ The paper used in this publication meets the minimum requirements of American National Standard for Information Sciences—Permanence of Paper for Printed Library Materials, ANSI/NISO Z39.48-1992.

Printed in the United States of America

Contents

List of Figures

List of Tables

Acknowledgments

We all occupy intersecting identities that reflect our many walks of life. I feel so lucky that I am a part of a vast village of support, love, and encouragement that enables me to find space and time to continue my creative and scholarly pursuits. I'd like to thank everyone in the village that helps me to raise my children and who walks with me in this rewarding life. These include my family, first and foremost. And I thank my children for the lovely people they are and the powerful force they are becoming. I especially thank our sitters and tutors, along with David Griffith, Keith Harris, and the Helm, Washington, and Gordon families, who grounded my support network during my travel to participate in the Safe Global Water Institute Summit and years following.

Secondly, I acknowledge the women, men, and children of East Africa who inspire us all. And I extend a huge debt of gratitude to the many scholars and activists who are pointing the way to solutions to the challenges of water and sanitation in East Africa. I also thank the University of Illinois Mandela Washington fellows from all over the African continent who participated in our Public Management Institute in 2016 and graciously provided feedback on ideas articulated in this manuscript.

Next, I thank my awesome co-editor, Dr. Brenda Sanya, and all authors and co-authors of the chapters in this volume. I am grateful to Dr. Sonali Ghosh, who did the careful footwork to populate our list of authors and find their university appointments and websites. And I appreciate Arianna Jenkins, Brian Pianfetti, Benito Marinas, Peter Luswata, Jeremy Guest, and the SGWI and 2013 summit participants for their rich insights.

I would not be at the University of Illinois if it were not for colleagues who contribute to a vibrant and inclusive intellectual environment resulting both from their scholarly contributions and from their interventions, such as Chancellor Robert Jones, vice provosts Abbas Benmamoun and Reitu Mabokela, Dean Wojtek Chodkzo-Zajko, and professors Antoinette Burton, Craig Koslofsky, Faye Harrison, Ruby Mendenhall, Kevin Hamilton, and Karen Flynn.

Institutional support from Illinois International Business Operations and the Center for African Studies, and especially Terri Gitler, Katrina Chester, and Cheryl Heck, has been indispensable. I also thank my administrative support staff: Lori Mikos for assistance to my educational equity work while I was a Graduate College associate dean and Mary Callaway and Andréa Fain for their assistance in my work at the Office of the Chancellor.

My intellectual village of support includes the insights offered by coauthors Biko Agozino, Marj DeVault, Mary Romero, and Michael O. West; colleagues at the Illinois Program for Research in the Humanities, the Center for African Studies, and the Departments of Sociology and Gender and Women's Studies; participants in our writing group; attenders at multiple conference sessions; and reviewers who have provided comments to book chapters in earlier formats.

I am grateful to Ms. Kathryn Tafelski, who believed in this work from the beginning, and to Emily Rodrick and the staff at Lexington Books and Rowman & Littlefield for their expert managing of the entire publication process. And finally, I thank Molly Bentsen for her tireless work to copy edit this manuscript. Her attention to detail and style are unsurpassed.

—Assata Zerai, editor

I would like to thank Assata Zerai for inviting me to join this exciting project, which allowed me to continue thinking critically about the ways in which the collisions and collusions of geopolitical changes, normativity, and economic imperatives order the lives of women and about how African feminisms and African women continue to reorder social life. I am thankful to Durell Callier, Malathi Iyengar, Cameron McCarthy, Anne N. Lutomia, and Karishma Desai for robust discussions on knowledge production and to Phantus W. Odero for his insights on social literacies and for the environmental and sustainable projects done by the African Youth Initiative on Climate Change–Kenya Chapter, among other organizations. Much of the qualitative research documented in the chapter "Public Goods, Citizenship Rights" was conducted as part of my research for an MA in gender/cultural studies. I am grateful to Dorothy Sanya Gautier, Donald E. Sanya, and Elizabeth Westvold for their support during the research project. Next I would like to thank Meiver De la Cruz, Crystal Rizzo, and Rama Srinivasan for reading my earliest drafts and my thesis advisor Sarah L. Leonard, as well as Carole Biewener, Laura Prieto, and Valerie Leiter, for insights that helped the development of this interdisciplinary work. I would also like to thank Theresa A. Perry for challenging me to consider the role of power in education and knowledge production as it emerged in the conversations among the women I spoke to and was echoed in policy papers. My deepest gratitude is to the women in Nyawara, who willingly shared such intimate stories about their lives. Finally, I would like to acknowledge Doris Wanyangu, Abner Sanya, and Abigail N. Sanya for their help in understanding how government policies, customary laws, education, and knowledge production have existed and continue to be transformed in local and national contexts in Kenya.

—Brenda N. Sanya, co-editor

Introduction

Assata Zerai and Brenda N. Sanya

The lives of women and children on the continent of Africa have been taken up as a subject of study by a host of notable researchers.[1] Working at times in integrated fashion, but often at odds with one another, activists, governmental and nongovernmental entities, and policymakers have pursued numerous interventions to improve health outcomes, educational prospects, and general well-being. Examples abound: from local groups, with or without national or international platforms (such as The African Youth Initiative on Climate Change, Stand with Eva, Warembo ni Yes, Uganda Housing Cooperative Union Limited [UHOCU], and Uganda Women's Efforts to Save Orphans [UWESO]), committed to making strides toward improving the lives of women and children; to national, regional, and transnational programs.[2] In the current iteration of Western influence in Africa, civil and environmental engineers[3] are taking up the charge to offer safe water and sanitation technologies to urban, periurban, and rural settings. Often missing from national and international discourse, and underutilized in intervention design, women's voices must come to the fore. Recognizing the multifaceted challenges to improving maternal and child health in East Africa, in this manuscript we unpack complex relationships among women's agency, access to water and sanitation, women's education and health literacy, and early childhood morbidity.

Through an African feminist lens we highlight the intricacies of deeply entrenched, yet fixable challenges experienced by women and children in East Africa seeking to access clean water and adequate sanitation and how the lack of uniform access to these necessities has gendered effects. The framework we offer will unveil inequities in the distribution of these resources in Kenya, Tanzania, and Uganda as well as paint a multilayered picture of the lives of women and girls, the predominant providers of water to households.

This work contributes to discussions and critiques of development effectiveness, to elucidations of African feminism and African feminist methodology, to our understanding of environmental contamination as an important determinant of maternal and child health (MCH), and to liberation studies of the postcolonial state. Demographic and Health Survey data from these three countries as well as qualitative data are analyzed.

WESTERN INFLUENCES

According to Africa Action, "We are faced with enormous barriers: . . . structural adjustment programs, driven by the World Bank and International Monetary Fund, destroy public health-care systems; and debt to rich countries hampers financing of vital social services, including health-care. Community mobilization and civil society action are essential for forcing action and ensuring greater accountability from all these institutions" (2007). This decade-old statement still well frames issues of concern.

We know that "globalization is a gendered phenomenon . . . [which] . . . positions and affects men and women differently, and . . . produces new forms of power and disadvantage" (Hawkesworth, 2006, p. 2). To more clearly understand "power and disadvantage" and how it differentially orders contemporary life in East Africa, colonialism, conquest, and capitalism must be understood not simply as historical moments or events that supplant cultures and lives of those who are colonized but as transformative processes that continue to be reproduced. In the North American context, J. Kēhaulani Kauanui (2016) and Beenash Jafri (2017), writing and thinking through Patrick Wolfe's "Settler Colonialism and the Elimination of the Native" (2006), have argued persuasively that the process of settler colonialism was not an event or moment in history, but that it can be "characterized as a structure, a system, and a logic" (Kauanui 2016) that continues to order, define, and subjugate the subjects it deems uncivil. This argument certainly resonates with the East African context based on global market dominance that orders geopolitical and socioeconomic policy decisions as well as (particularly in the Kenyan case) the role of the transformed structure where white settlers as well as transnational nongovernmental agencies shape policy and multinational corporations drive decision making regarding the privatization of public goods and infrastructure development.

Colonial government policy in East Africa, which worked alongside religious missions, was pervasive. Beginning with churches, missionary hospitals, and schools, East Africans encountered pervasive, unified government and church policies that entrenched administrative and settler colonial rule, which translated governmental policies into institutional practices that centered "civilization" and acculturation interactions that required civilization processes. And even though East Africans were not passive recipients of the mutually constitutive projects of Western religion, education, and governance, Enlightenment reasoning took hold. The promises of Enlightenment, such as modernization, progress, and universalism, were taught in schools, enforced by governments, provided by health care and social service providers, and celebrated in religiosity tied to colonial structures of government. The lingering effects of colonialism and the effects of contemporary economic structures thus are still raced, gendered, and classed, differentially cast in different locations; education, as a colonial product, was and is still contingent upon and in service of "material and symbolic economies of modern capitalism that demand land theft, extraction, and labor exploitation for the accumulation of ruling class wealth" (Angod 2015, p. 428). The introduction of contemporary sanitation and water distribution methods in East Africa, as part of the civilizing mission, furthered the Western agenda of progress and of capitalism's demands[4] by "gently teach[ing] Third World Others about civility" (Razack 2004, p. 33).

For instance, under British colonial rule of Kenya, the education of Black and South Asian children was in place to reinforce national hierarchies and make recipients "civilized," subservient subjects of the colonial government. The unified government policy that took root in social life was reinforced through targeted health, sanitation, and educational policies underscored in various spheres. For the majority of Black students, education emphasized technical training and basic literacy skills to produce teachers for Black schools and clerks to translate and transmit policies of the colonial administration. Educated Black Kenyans quickly realized the long-term objectives and effects of this racial stratification witnessed in education. By 1925, there were protests that education was distributed in uneven ways. For instance, rural vocational training, responsible for educating most Black students, was not academically rigorous, and it focused on farming and industrial education, while a select few Black and Asian students and all White students received classical liberal arts education that addressed and emphasized major issues facing students, their communities, and colonial Kenya. The contradiction was obvious: on the one hand, education was positioned as the key to economic and social progress; on the other hand, the social relations of Western liberalism excluded colonized people through educational opportunities that instituted and normalized hierarchies across the nation. Put simply, even though some schools provided rigorous educational opportunities, these schools had limited pupil spaces and were focused on the acculturation to British norms, social practices, and forms of governance. Education within schools linked to economic and social progress is described in national policy as success, as discussed in chapter 3 ("Public Goods, Citizenship Rights"). Over time, these norms and practices didn't function as advances; rather, they remained impositions. Moreover, the introduction of Western-centric social services, as part of a unified civilizing project, was poorly implemented, disrupted cultural norms, and eventually became unsustainable and upended existing practices that have been used successfully. This introduction of Western schooling, judicial processes, infrastructure, education, health care services, and widespread policies hinges upon a normalization of the structures of colonialism, including the introduction of systems that were unsustainable and continue to fail. However, the failure of those policies is rarely interrogated in development studies that focus less on the lingering structures, effects, and failure of colonial conquest and more on what are considered uncivilized local traditions. In such models of development, integration into global markets and cultures means that neocolonial structures take on colonial practices and make them contemporary policies and practices.

This turn away from local innovation toward Western models bypasses the feasibility of sustainable policies seeking to address water and sanitation concerns.[5] Some influences from the West today are positive or helpful to many families in East Africa, but many of the problems that exist in Africa today were created or exacerbated under colonialism. Capitalist "malevolence of colonial accumulation" (Nyong'o 2007) and West-centric development practiced for the past 500 years (Behrendt 2008) have undermined indigenous efforts to ensure access to safe water and have destroyed epistemologies of waste throughout the continent of Africa (van Vliet et al. 2014). A timeline that begins from incursion into Africa from the West circa 1514, as introduced in chapter 2, demonstrates that Western influence was largely detrimental. The historical and contemporary factors that have led to the maldistribution of safe water and sanitation infrastructure in East Africa, such as the division between women's work (including shifting cultivation, subsistence farming, and food production) and men's work (settled, plow-based cultivation and private land tenure), remain as part of the colonial heritage of British imperialism, the contemporary influences of multinational corporations, and the economic structural adjustment programs that continue to shape policymaking. Not only did the West depopulate the coastal areas during the transatlantic slave trade, but it continued to depopulate (Caldwell 1985) and dehumanize Africans remaining on the continent through colonialism and settler colonialism (Rodney 1981). Indigenous technologies for protecting water sources and disposing of waste were disrupted and destroyed as a result of Western interference (White 2002; Muyambo and Maposa 2014).

The technologies that replaced indigenous practices were focused on providing services to settler populations (Okia 2012, van Vliet et al. 2014), the vast majority living in what are now urban areas. This led to the uneven development we see in East Africa to this day. So, for example, only 25% of households in Kenya have drinking water piped to the residence (into the home or in the yard). But in urban areas the percentage more than doubles: 56% of households in urban Kenya have drinking water piped to the residence (Kenya National Bureau of Statistics and ICF Macro 2010). In Tanzania, the differences are even greater. There, only 8% of households have water piped into residences, whereas in urban areas it is 19% (Tanzania Central Statistical Office and Institute for Resource Development/Macro Systems 2010). And in Uganda only 6.4% have water piped into residences compared with four times as many—28%—in urban areas (Uganda Bureau of Statistics and Institute for Resource Development/Macro Systems 2011). These cleavages have improved over time, but those established hundreds of years ago remain.

Another aspect of West-centric capitalist development in East Africa that contributes to inequitable access to safe water and sanitation is the role of multinational entities, including the exploitation of workers and natural resources (Nyong'o 1988), concomitant with the creation of development products such as roads, railways, and airports in service of corporate interests rather than the interests of countries' citizens (Langdon 1974, Weintstein 2008). Progress, innovation, and distribution of water and sanitation services have been defined on Western (and global economic) terms and defined by an almost singular goal of creating wealth. It is in this framework that Kenya introduced "Vision 2030" (Government of the Republic of Kenya 2007), a national strategic plan to position Kenya "towards a globally competitive and prosperous nation." The Vision 2030 policy on water and sanitation ("To ensure Water and Improved Sanitation availability and access to all by 2030") addresses five areas: water resource management, water harvesting and storage, water supply, sanitation, and irrigation and drainage. The policy focuses extensively on management, harvesting, and distribution of water, and the policy recommendations focus on infrastructural development, improved sanitation and hygiene awareness, and a capital investment in irrigation schemes. The loans provided by the World Bank and International Monetary Fund (IMF) and the economic structural adjustment programs (ESAP) imposed are influences wielded by multinational corporations, leading to uneven development (Weintstein 2008; *Daily Monitor* 2012).

The tourism industry is another influence on West-centric development (Rotarou 2014). In Tanzania, for example, water piped into residences is much more available on the island of Zanzibar—with high tourist development—than on the mainland (31% of Zanzibar households have water piped in residences, almost four times that of the rest of the country). The inequitable distribution of clean water and safe sanitation infrastructure has implications for social justice in these settings, and responsibility for this injustice is the result of historical injustices meted by Western influences as well as present-day practices.

SOCIAL JUSTICE FRAMEWORK

Social justice advocacy describes efforts to increase fairness in the distribution of resources; end discrimination against all groups, fostering values that recognize all people as equal; and promote both the participation of people in policy and implementation processes affecting their lives and transparency and accountability for how decisions are made and how those decisions affect society (Klugman 2011). Clearly, better water and sanitation would help social justice because it would increase fairness in the distribution of this crucial resource to target communities in East Africa.[6]

In regards to gender equity, one way the lack of sanitation in East African settings affects women is by making them vulnerable. Notably, in the Kibera, the largest low-income informal housing settlement, located in Nairobi, Kenya, sanitation facilities are woefully inadequate. Amnesty International (2010) reports that it is common that pit latrines, shared by more than 100 people, require for most residents a 10-minute walk or more. This not only increases environmental contamination from improper alternative methods of disposing of human waste, such as "flying toilets" (plastic bags filled with feces, tied closed, and discarded), but it adds to violence and insecurity, especially of female residents and children.

The safety concerns for women that arise when they lack access to adequate toilet facilities on their premises is a concern in all of our research sites. In a World Bank Report, the authors note that "women who lack sanitation often risk sexual harassment on the way to and from their defecation site. . . . The emancipation that a latrine (on their premises) bestows on such women cannot lightly be dismissed" (Cairncross and Valdmanis 2006).

While most discourses surrounding so-called flying toilets in Kenya have provided a trenchant critique of the environmental concerns, failed sanitation services, and cultural taboos about discussing toilets and toilet use, there is little conversation that flying toilets are perhaps a response to safety concerns in addition to a lack of facilities and education. The intimate connection between vulnerability, corruption, and disadvantage functions to limit resource distribution; the sanitation, health, and environmental concerns, like corruption,

> violates the rights of all those affected [. . . however . . .] it has a disproportionate impact on people that belong to groups that are exposed to particular risks (such

> as minorities, indigenous peoples, migrant workers, disabled people, those with HIV/AIDS, refugees, prisoners and those who are poor). It also disproportionately affects women and children. (Sahu 2012, p. 71)

Even the education of children and adults is affected by lack of access to safe water at their residence. This is so because females, including girl children, are responsible for carrying water to provide it to the household. So in Kenya, for example, for most households it takes 30 minutes or more to fetch water (from analysis of Demographic and Health Survey [DHS] data). In 76% of households, women fetch water; in 5% of households, girls under the age of 15 fetch water (analysis of DHS data for 2009). This takes many hours a day and affects girls' educational access. The Arusha Region in Tanzania offers another example: in 46% of households, members travel up to 30 minutes to get drinking water; another 45% have to travel more than 30 minutes.

An association also exists between sanitation and education. Safe sanitation in schools would likely increase girls' safety in schools and improve health outcomes so that children miss fewer school days. Improved long-term health outcomes would lead to lower stunting and wasting of children (Smith et al. 2013; Humphrey 2009; Zerai 2014) and better physical and mental development so that they can better retain what they learn in school. In this case, it would also improve education of adults over the long run because the improved sanitation of children and the resulting improvements in education would likely improve future life chances when the children become adults.

SANITATION AND QUALITY OF LIFE

Currently sanitation resources are woefully inadequate in East Africa, where in Kenya only 7.5% of households have unshared flush toilets (Kenya National Bureau of Statistics [KNBS] and ICF Macro 2010), in Tanzania only 10% (Tanzania Central Statistical Office and Institute for Resource Development/Macro Systems 2010), and in Uganda a tiny 1.8% (Uganda Bureau of Statistics and Institute for Resource Development/Macro Systems 2011). Urban areas in all three countries have better access to flush toilets, but even there the resource is not distributed evenly. In Nairobi, for example, where 34% of households overall have access to unshared flush toilets (Kenya National Bureau of Statistics [KNBS] and ICF Macro 2010), the neighboring informal settlement area of Kibera, boasting over a million residents (Amnesty International 2010) has very little access to clean water and safe sanitation. "One in four households have access to a toilet, forcing residents to share pit latrines with an average of 50 other people" (Rousselot 2010). In Kibera, toilet facilities and improved drainage are named the top health priorities by 60% of women; toilet facilities, drainage, and safe water are named by 75% (African Population and Health Research Center 2002). In Tanzania, 65% of households use open pit/pit latrine without slab, and 14% have no toilet facilities (Tanzania Central Statistical Office [CSO] and Institute for Resource Development/Macro Systems 2016). In urban Uganda over half of households share total facilities, and 28% do not enjoy improved facilities. Overall, 75% in Uganda lack access to improved facilities, so they have either no toilet facilities or an open pit without a slab.

AFRICAN FEMINIST FRAMEWORK/METHODOLOGY

A capitalist West-centric problem requires an African woman–centered perspective for critique, analysis, and family-focused solutions. Engineers, development specialists, humanitarians, charity-based entities, and those who sincerely wish to offer acceptable and appropriate solutions to issues such as water and sanitation offer technological know-how, but they all can benefit from social science contributions regarding how to create bottom-up solutions that will not inadvertently reproduce inequality.

We approach the study of safe water and sanitation in East Africa from the perspectives of environmental sociology,[7] African feminist studies,[8] and critical postcolonial studies.[9] The lens of African feminist studies, an important branch of and often even a corrective to second-wave feminism and postcolonial studies, helps us to address the social contexts among women and children in East Africa as well as to unveil their underlying social structures from the colonial period through 2011. We extend and test the hypothesis that West-centric development (as characterized by uneven development focused on urban areas, as a remnant of its colonial past, and by economic structural adjustment policies, a current neoliberal reality) in East Africa has deleterious effects on safe water and sanitation with significant effects on young children's health. To examine this, we describe the ways we see these dominant influences built into the underlying social structure of these societies, as a result of East Africa's colonial past and the uneven distribution of development resources.

To address a capitalist West-centric problem we apply an African woman–centered perspective for critique, analysis, and family-focused solutions, given that it is at the intersection of social categorizations, power structures, political forces that people make crucial decisions about their everyday health, families, lives, and futures. Moreover, such an analysis must be local and not universal, as Nkiru Nzegwu (2004) argues: "False universalization of the Western concept of woman [. . .] highlights the intrusive nature of the Western metaphysics of gender on theoretical formulations in and about other cultures" (p. 1), as womanhood in relationship to masculinity does not map out universally. Taking heed from Nzegwu's intervention we understand gender, first, as having multiple categories and, second, that within those multiple categories, understanding hierarchies demands an understanding of power structures.

Building upon the work of African/Africana feminist researchers, including humanists and social scientists on the African continent and in the African diaspora—such as Micere Mugo (1991), Oyèrónkẹ́ Oyěwùmí (1997, 2003, 2005), Teresa Barnes (2013), Amina Mama (2002), Patricia Hill Collins (1986, 1990, 1998), Elsa Barkley Brown (1995), Audre Lorde (1984), Michael West (2002, 2005), Biko Agozino (1999), Mary Osirim (2003), Horace Campbell (2003), and others—we will explore a framework that considers the ways that gender, class, neocolonial relations (Imam and Mama 1994), ethnicity/race, religion, nation, sexuality, globalization, and other dimensions of oppression intersect to impact the experiences and agency of individuals and groups attempting to access safe water and sanitation in East Africa. As in previous work (Zerai 2014), we propose an *African feminist* scientific methodology that derives from feminist frameworks, especially from African feminisms.[10]

The African feminist framework and its intersectional analysis considers how the matrix of domination and interlocking spheres of oppression (Collins 1990) affect African women and children simultaneously. It exposes and opens up our understanding of the ways these forces operate, better revealing the underlying structures of society. This helps us to place the phenomena of water, sanitation, and children's health in East Africa in relevant social, political, economic, and cultural context. It guides our exploration of how spheres of nation, class, gender, ethnicity, and sexuality operate simultaneously and proposes relationships among these various social forces.

We examine the institutional factors, community conditions, access to water and sanitation, and family-level behavioral factors influencing early childhood morbidity in postcolonial East Africa. Our principal evidence is derived from analyses of the Demographic and Health Survey data sets collected by each country's own Ministry of Health, MACRO-International, and the U.S. Agency for International Development. Further, survey and qualitative data gathered by co-authors aid our ability to offer a unique perspective.

THE CHALLENGE

We argue for an African feminist analysis to address decolonial practices in improving health, water distribution, and sanitation. In the past, "issues of national production or reproduction [have] not relate[d] to women, but instead to state bureaucrats or intellectuals" (Yuval-Davis 1997, p. 22). The hidden nature of women's contribution can in part be attributed to the social contract model of statecraft on which most states continue to be founded and which distinguishes between the public and private spheres. Women and the family are circumscribed to the private domain and are not seen as politically relevant. "[T]he exclusion of women from [the public domain] . . . has contributed to their exclusion from this discourse as well" (Okech 2011, p. 54). From this perspective, our objective is to evaluate how the exclusion of women from policy discussions and design of implementation strategies on improving safe water and sanitation and ultimately on child health outcomes impacts households and communities in East Africa. While the people of East Africa have asked the relevant questions when assessing their countries' development—namely, "What has been happening to poverty? What has been happening to unemployment? What has been happening to inequality?" (Seers 1969)—we ask, "Where are the women?" (Shoeman 2004).

Social development in East Africa has not taken place in a vacuum. Its outer context is a world market economy. Though consumed by the need to become a middle-income economy, East Africa has a disadvantaged position in the world market economy, subordinated to more economically developed countries that wield power in the world market by limiting imports from less economically developed countries (LDCs), by paying less for imports, or by charging more for exports to LDCs. Richer countries can buffer their own economic crises by burdening LDCs (Rodney 1981). Economic volatility is endemic to LDCs because of their economically and politically disadvantaged positions. State corruption has benefited from these external forces and has further crippled East Africa's economies.

East Africa has endured multiple challenges to lowering early childhood morbidity in recent years, including but not limited to economic volatility, malaria, the HIV/AIDS crisis, political instability, the global financial crisis, and climate change. In light of these difficulties faced by countries, especially in the Global South, in September 2015 the United Nations General Assembly formally adopted the 2030 Agenda for Sustainable Development, operationalized as 17 Sustainable Development Goals "to transform our world" (United Nations 2015).

Sustainable Development Goals

State officials, in cooperation with medical practitioners, families, and other stakeholders, are working to improve the conditions of poor children in the world. UN sustainable development goals (SDGs) call for improved access to water and sanitation and reduction in early childhood morbidity by 2030.

Formerly designated as millennium development goals (MDGs), the goals act as a mechanism to improve accountability, reenergize commitment, and recognize successes (United Nations 2008). The 2030 Agenda for Sustainable Development (United Nations 2015, p. 3–4) includes multiple indicators of progress. The goals follow.

1. End poverty in all its forms everywhere.
2. End hunger, achieve food security and improved nutrition and promote sustainable agriculture.
3. Ensure healthy lives and promote well-being for all at all ages.
4. Ensure inclusive and equitable quality education and promote lifelong learning opportunities for all.
5. Achieve gender equality and empower all women and girls.
6. Ensure availability and sustainable management of water and sanitation for all.
7. Ensure access to affordable, reliable, sustainable and modern energy for all.
8. Promote sustained, inclusive and sustainable economic growth, full and productive employment and decent work for all.
9. Build resilient infrastructure, promote inclusive and sustainable industrialization and foster innovation.
10. Reduce inequality within and among countries.
11. Make cities and human settlements inclusive, safe, resilient and sustainable.
12. Ensure sustainable consumption and production patterns.
13. Take urgent action to combat climate change and its impacts.
14. Conserve and sustainably use the oceans, seas and marine resources for sustainable development.
15. Protect, restore and promote sustainable use of terrestrial ecosystems, sustainably manage forests, combat desertification, and halt and reverse land degradation and halt biodiversity loss.
16. Promote peaceful and inclusive societies for sustainable development, provide access to justice for all and build effective, accountable and inclusive institutions at all levels.
17. Strengthen the means of implementation and revitalize the global partnership for sustainable development.

In a 2016 assessment, Lim et al. examine health-related SDGs in 188 countries. They find Kenya ranked 146th, Tanzania 154th, and Uganda 173rd (all in the bottom quarter of countries examined) for what they identify as a health-related SDG index, which takes into account stunting, wasting, under-5 mortality, maternal mortality, water/sanitation and hygiene mortality, and other factors. Here we focus on young children because of their vulnerability to inadequate water and sanitation resources. SDG indicators include improved nutrition, improving women's status, and access to safe drinking water and sanitation.

> Globally, in 2014, nearly 1 in 4 children under the age of 5, an estimated total of 159 million children, had stunted growth. Stunting is defined as inadequate height for age, an indicator of the cumulative effects of undernutrition and infection. Southern Asia and subSaharan Africa accounted for three quarters of the children under 5 with stunted growth in 2014. (United Nations 2017)

According to Lim et al. (2016), the median stunting prevalence of children under age 5 in the 188 countries measured was 12.5%, with a minimum of 0 and a maximum of 54.5%. Only 16.5% of countries had already achieved the SDG target by 2015. In the East African countries under examination, Kenya is in the 63rd percentile in regard to stunting, Tanzania the 45th, and Uganda the 55th. In terms of unsafe and unimproved water and sanitation resources, Kenya was in the 25th and 24th percentiles, Tanzania the 24th and 11th percentiles, and Uganda the 26th and 20th percentiles, respectively. So all three countries were in the bottom quarter for water and sanitation resources, with Tanzania an outlier in the bottom 11% of countries in access to safe and improved sanitation.

AN AFRICAN FEMINIST AND VINDICATIONIST-TRANSCONTINENTAL PERSPECTIVE

We use an African feminist methodology and insights from African feminism to determine our empirical and analytic tools. We foreground feminist and women-centered intellectual work that emanates from East Africa, including that of Adeleke Adeeko, Lisa Aubrey, Tabitha Kanogo, Micere Mugo, Keguro Macharia, Evan Maina Mwangi, Dorothy Mbilinyi, Wambui Mwangi, George Odhiambo, Sylvia Tamale, Awino Okech, Stella Nyanzi, L. Muthoni Wanyeki, Shailja Patel, Grace Musila, Anne Lutomia, Kerubo Abuya, Dorothy Rombo and so many others. African feminism is an appropriate perspective from which to assess new technologies in African settings (Zerai 2014). Amina Mama articulates African feminism well in her editorial of the inaugural issue of *Feminist Africa: Intellectual Politics* (Nov/Dec 2002, Issue 1, 150):

> African gender politics have become increasingly complex and contradictory. Feminism, as a movement that is both global and local, leaves little untouched. In postcolonial contexts it presents a praxis that directly opposes the hegemonic interests of multinational corporations, international financial and development

> agencies and nation states as well as the persisting male domination of disparate traditional structures, civil society formations and social movements. . . . African women are mobilizing at local, regional and international levels, and deploying various strategies and forms.

According to Imam, Mama, and Sow, "engendering African social science is not a simple development of knowledge, but is also necessarily and simultaneously profoundly a political struggle over power and resources" (1997, p. 2). They argue that "social science which does not acknowledge gender as an analytic category is an impoverished and distorted science, and cannot accurately explain social realities and hence cannot provide a way out of the present crisis in Africa" (p. 2).

Considerations for African feminist methodology to be used in analyzing the success of safe water and sanitation technologies include the following (as cited in Zerai 2014):

- Inclusion of all African women in data analyses, as well as centering women who would otherwise be marginalized, identifying multiple and simultaneous oppressions, and recognizing women's agency.
- Analysis of women's experiences in context by considering macroeconomic, political, and social factors and identifying relations of power.
- Multilevel analysis that interrogates individual-level variables by exploring analytic constructs and identifying contextual factors such as maternal education levels in the community, health resources available to communities, and community infrastructure.
- Transparency in research perspectives and objectives and consistency with national liberation and progressive social change.
- Identification of the subject of study in ways that ring true to women in the setting, so that their interests drive research agendas, creating research that is African-centered and woman-centered.
- Production of knowledge that has clear policy relevance to improve lives on the ground.
- Work to ensure that new technologies introduced to better the lives of individuals in the community are implemented in a way that considers their impact upon women and children and that does not exacerbate existing inequalities.

This last consideration is much more focused on application, and we must introduce this feature into African feminist analysis in order to positively impact social policy and its products.

Further, we distinguish this work as that falling within the tradition that Bill Martin and Michael West have identified as "vindicationist/transcontinentalism." They argue that "the vindicationist tradition (so labeled by the late St. Clair

Drake) was primarily historical, encompassing the great African kingdoms and civilizations in North as well as West Africa" (1999, p. 86). It "had its origins in attempts by Black intellectuals, writers, pamphleteers and memorialists to vindicate Africa and Africans, to defend them against their traducers in Europe and the Americas who hurled calumnies about a 'Dark Africa' devoid of history and culture. Vindicationism, in brief, was a project to negate the 'whiting out' of the African past" (p. 87). Martin and West note that a fundamental characteristic of vindicationist scholarship was its transnational and transcontinental perspective. Its adherents connected ancient Africa to modern Africa, Africa north of the Sahara to Africa south of the Sahara, and especially the African continent to the African diaspora. They tended to concentrate on the broad political, religious, and cultural themes that transcended national and continental boundaries in the Black world. These hallmarks of 19th-century vindicationism continued well into the 20th century to inform the work of professionally trained Black scholars, including Carter G. Woodson, W. E. B Du Bois, and William Leo Hansberry.

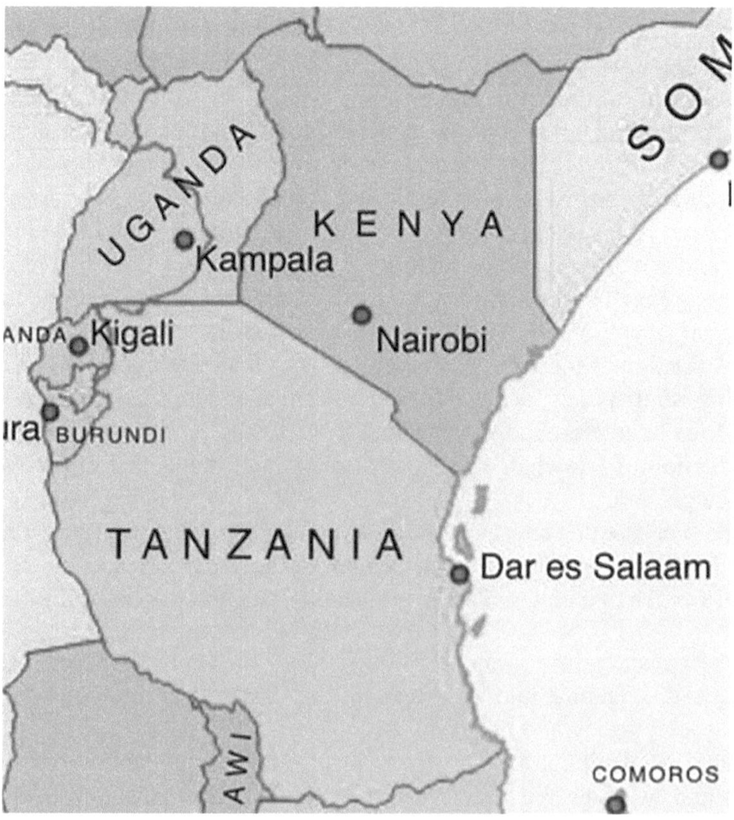

Figure 0.1. Map of East Africa (Kenya, Tanzania, Uganda)
mapswire.com

We align our perspectives of the study of safe water and sanitation in East Africa within the vindicationalist/transcontinental tradition.[11]

The East African Community Development Strategy

The East African Community (EAC 2001, EAC 2016) has been in existence since 1999.

> The Vision of EAC is a prosperous, competitive, secure, stable and politically united East Africa; and the mission is to widen and deepen Economic, Political, Social and Culture integration in order to improve the quality of life of the people of East Africa through increased competitiveness, value added production, trade and investments.

The founding member states are Kenya, United Republic of Tanzania, and Uganda. Since the organization's founding, other partner states, notably the Republic of Rwanda and the Republic of Burundi, have joined EADC (see Figure 0.1).

THE CHAPTERS

In this introduction, we have described the context of our study. We have distinguished our work by placing it squarely in an African feminist vindicationist tradition, and we have explained our choice of East Africa as a site for understanding water, sanitation, and children's health. In chapter 1 we explore the lives of women and children there. Focusing on historical and social characteristics of East Africa, we end the chapter by examining a day in the lives of women in various social locations and how water and sanitation shape their daily experiences and those of their children. In chapter 2, Shorma Bianca Bailey and Assata Zerai explain historical and contemporary factors that have led to the maldistribution of safe water and sanitation infrastructure in East Africa. The factors include the uneven development instigated as part of the region's colonial heritage, the influences of multinational corporations, economic structural adjustment programs, the tourism industry, failing development infrastructure, and the incursion of nongovernmental organizations (NGOs). In chapter 3, Brenda N. Sanya examines how the confluence of colonialism and patriarchy defines rural women's access to health, and we explore the perils of an assumption that education is always directly linked to schooling and that it is emancipatory. Rejecting the idea that education (the process of receiving instruction at an institution) is always emancipatory, we show how existing indigenous and customary systems of learning can provide solutions that are relevant to improving the lives of women. In chapter 4, on the basis of analysis of survey data and government documents, Teresia R. Olemako examines the river basin model of water governance in the Kilimanjaro region of Tanzania. In chapter 5, Assata Zerai and Rebecca L. Morrow use the lens of gender to analyze new technologies to improve access to safe, drinkable water and adequate sanitation in African countries. In chapter 6, Assata Zerai, Rebecca L. Morrow, and Courtney Cuthbertson analyze effects of water and sanitation on early childhood morbidity and illustrate the importance of intranational variation in levels of development for child health outcomes. And in the conclusion, Assata Zerai and Joanna B. Perez summarize policy recommendations concerning current and proposed water and sanitation interventions offered in the book and delineate the scholarship of women in Kenya, Tanzania, and Uganda. We evaluate these in light of East African women's scholarship and propose future intellectual endeavors.

NOTES

1. Some include Cuthbert Omari, Emmah Gweshi, Sylvia Tamale, Relebohile Moletsane, Stella Nyanzi, Ama Ata Aido, Omofolabo Ajayi-Soyinka, Oyèrónkẹ́ Oyěwùmí, Judith A. Byfield, Neelika Jayawardane, Michere Mugo, Wambui Mwangi, Rudo Gaidzanwa, Amina Mama, Teresa Barnes, Toyin Falola, the late Elaine Salo, and Paul Farmer.

2. Recent examples: Slum Dwellers International; Tanzania Gender Networking Programme; the Feminist Activist Coalition (FemAct in Tanzania); National Network of Farmers Group in Tanzania (Mviwata); President Barack Obama, who pledged $7 billion in aid for power infrastructure in 2013; Michelle Obama's work with the U.S. Peace Corps Let Girls Learn program; President Jimmy Carter, whose foundation led in reducing Guinea worm disease from 3.5 million cases in 1986 to 25 in 2016 and promotes the rights of women and girls; the World Health Organization; the Clinton Health Initiative; and the Bill and Melinda Gates Foundation, contributing to successes bringing down the number of HIV infections and increasing percentages receiving treatment worldwide. Even entertainers have been involved, such as Oprah Winfrey, founder of a leadership academy in South Africa; and Bono, contributor to campaigns to raise money for HIV treatment and prevention in the global south and for the eradication of extreme poverty.

3. Notable projects are the Water Campus at the University of Illinois, which is heavily involved with creating appropriate water and sanitation technologies in East Africa; and the Water, Health and Development research program at Stanford University, Woods Institute for the Environment.

4. Federici (2004, p. 17) writes of capitalism's breadth: [C]apitalism, as a social-economic system, is necessarily committed to racism and sexism. For capitalism must justify and mystify the contradictions built into its social relations—the promise

of freedom vs. the reality of widespread coercion, and the promise of prosperity vs. the reality of widespread penury—by denigrating the "nature" of those it exploits: women, colonial subjects, the descendants of African slaves, the immigrants displaced by globalization. At the core of capitalism there is not only the symbiotic relation between waged contractual labor and enslavement but, together with it, the dialectics of accumulation and destruction of labor-power, for which women have paid the highest cost, with their bodies, their work, their lives. It is impossible therefore to associate capitalism with any form of liberation or attribute the longevity of the system to its capacity to satisfy human needs. If capitalism has been able to reproduce itself it is only because of the web of inequalities that it has built into the body of the world proletariat and because of its capacity to globalize exploitation. This process is still unfolding under our eyes as it has for the last 500 years.

Inclusion into these systems does not transform the system; rather, it spreads the control of the system to include previously excluded populations.

5. For instance, introducing indoor plumbing and toilets in areas where water is scarce or plumbing extends through terrain that is unmonitored, while successful in urban areas and in the West, introduced challenges with no simple solutions for rural communities, which had long used and maintained outdoor and indoor pit latrines. Another contemporary example is the turn to Western processed foods, which has led to a different form of malnutrition being experienced in wealthy communities, including a rise in heart disease and obesity. This has quickly been followed by the return to "organic" food by the middle class as a Western development–driven model that exists side by side with communities that have always eaten organic foods.

6. Linking to the previous discussion of *How Europe Underdeveloped Africa* (Rodney 1981), some have called for reparations as compensation for stolen lives and land. In this moment, however, resources must be required in a way that helps to carry out national and local strategic visions for infrastructural investments.

7. Some authors writing in this tradition include Bair and Cayleff 1993; Charmaz 1991; Charmaz and Paterniti 1999; Conrad and Leiter 2003; Diamond 1992; Harding 1987; Harding and Norberg 2005; and Krieger and Fee 1994.

8. Herein "African" usage captures people of African descent, both those living on the continent of Africa and those living outside. I elaborate on its meaning in the section on U.S. Black studies. Others include Amadiume 1987, 1997; Brown 1995; Chepyator-Thomson 2005; Davis 1981, 1990; Qunta 1987; Steady 1985; Terborg-Penn and Rushing 1996; and Zinn et al. 1986.

9. Some include Alexander and Mohanty 1997; Freeman 2001; Henderson 2004; Mackintosh and Tibandebage 2006; Molyneux 2006; and Mwanza 1992.

10. The African feminist methodology utilized is not about "gender separatism." It instead highlights the need to ensure that women's voices are considered in social scientific and development agendas. For a fuller discussion of African feminism and African womanism and the ways African feminist methodology draws from both, see Zerai 2014.

11. For more details, see the Martin and West publication (1999).

Chapter One

The Lives of Women and Children in East Africa

Assata Zerai

Development resources in East Africa exist in the context of social, economic, political, and demographic change resulting from its traditional African heritages, Arab-Islamic rule, European-Christian dominance (Du Bois 1965; Nkrumah 1963; Caldwell 1985), independence movements, and postindependence life. The most important effects of these forces in East Africa are evident in push factors promoting health emanating from traditional practices to promote environmental sustainability and traditional birth practices such as midwifery, but these are coupled with pull factors detracting from development, including vestiges of colonialism, evident in extreme social inequality along class, racial, and ethnic lines and especially in the privileging of elites at home and abroad. This occurs both in terms of providing better access to improved water and sanitation for elite communities in-country and in facilitating multinational corporations' incursions into privatizing land and natural resources in exchange for kickbacks to national elites, while ordinary citizens are prevented from enjoying the fruits that natural resources and built technology could provide. So, doubletalk happens: development experts and their industrial partners speak of improved water, sanitation, and health while the reality on the ground is that women, men, and children too often languish in communities with inadequate access to the basic necessities of life.

I provide a brief overview of historical influences on the lives of women and children in East Africa, with a focus on Kenya, Tanzania and Uganda and explain a framework that summarizes the macroeconomic, political, and social factors that set the stage for living conditions related to water, sanitation, and ultimate child health outcomes (Zerai 2014). The framework covers four time periods: colonialism; independence movements; postindependence economic prosperity; and, varying by country, political destabilization, recession, and breakdown in development infrastructure (see Tables 1.1, 1.2, and 1.3). Finally, utilizing data from countries' Demographic and Health Surveys (2011) and other qualitative sources, I discuss everyday experiences impacting various sectors of women and girls in each setting.

DELIVERING ON THE PROMISES OF LIBERATION STRUGGLES

Tables 1.1, 1.2, and 1.3 provide an overview of the major factors that may contribute to health outcomes in early childhood. An important narrative and motivator that prompted popular involvement in independence movements was the promise of health, education, and equitable distribution of development resources to all citizens. Fluctuations in infant and child mortality rates, from immediately before independence to the latest available data, signal that some missteps have happened. A question posed by some students of this history is this: Do "all liberation struggles eventually end in betrayal"?[1] As shown below, postcolonial delivery on the promises made by liberation struggles' leadership has been complicated by many factors.

Statistics have little value unless they are understood in the contexts of the social worlds that produce them. I provide a brief overview of the economic, political, and social circumstances that precede and surround the current state of child health in East Africa. To guide this overview, I use frameworks that place child morbidity and mortality statistics in context (Tables 1.1, 1.2, and 1.3). I focus on the macro factors (column 1) and community conditions (column 2) that affect death of children under the age of 5 (under-5 mortality rate) because early childhood mortality is more greatly affected by poor social development and infrastructure. I focus on child mortality instead of growth stunting because anthropometric measures needed to provide growth-faltering data were not gathered in all rounds of the Demographic and Health Surveys (DHS), the primary data used for this discussion, and they are rarely gathered in national surveys. These health outcome data are shown in column 3 of Tables 1.1, 1.2 and 1.3. For statistics that harken back to periods before DHS data became available, and as far back as preindependence, I utilize estimates from the United Nations Children's Fund (UNICEF). I use the lower confidence boundary for most, as that data is generally more closely aligned with DHS data. Timelines with more detail are listed in Tables 1.4, 1.5, and 1.6.

Table 1.1. Kenya's History of Child Health, 1950–2014

[1] Macroeconomic, Political and Social Factors	➔	*[2] Community Conditions*	➔	*[3] Health Outcome*
PERIOD I (pre-1963) Colonial Era		– Colonial violence – Disenfranchisement of African populations – Inequitably distributed development infrastructure – Poor water and sanitation – Impoverishment in monetized economy – Prenatal and postnatal care inadequate – Few rural health centers – Railroad from Mombasa to Lake Victoria + Liberation movement + Traditional birth practitioners and herbalists	 1950: 1963:	*High* under-5 mortality CMR* 383–268/1,000 CMR 169–198/1,000 (high and low estimates indicated)
		Period II Contextual Considerations 🡓		
PERIOD II (1964–1989) Political independence and change in health policy		+ Free and compulsory education + Family planning education + Land reform measures, including improving water and sanitation in rural areas + Drought feeding programs + Free health care to majority + Prenatal care program + Rural primary health care centers built + Women's literacy and formal education – 1987 Opposition groups suppressed – 1977–89 Upward trend in under-5 growth faltering	1964: 1972: 1989:	Lowered child mortality CMR 164/1,000 CMR 136/1,000 CMR 91/1,000

(continued)

Table 1.1. *(Continued)*

[1] Macroeconomic, Political and Social Factors	→	*[2] Community Conditions*	→	*[3] Health Outcome*
		Period III Contextual Consideration ↓		
PERIOD III (1989–2003) Third and fourth decades of nationhood: corruption, ethnic tensions; World Bank withholds $5b; rent battles		– 1992 Ethnic conflict kills 2,000 + 1997 Demonstrations for democratic reform – 1997 World Bank withholds $5b in credit – 2001 Rent battles in Kibera + 2001 Parliament votes to import less-expensive HIV antiviral medications –/+ 1997 and 2002 elections – Masaai and Samburu groups accept $7m – 2000 Economic hardship; IMF suspends lending – 2003 Under-5 growth faltering: 15.8% + 2003 IMF resumes lending	 1993: 1998: 2003:	Increasing under-5 mortality CMR 93/1,000 CMR 105/1,000 CMR 113/1,000
		Period IV Contextual Considerations ↓		
PERIOD IV (2004–2014) Fifth decade of nationhood		– 2004–12 Corruption ensues – 2004/2006/2008 Food crises – 2005 Land and water rights clashes – 35,000 Somali refugees in Kenya – 2006–08 Elections Violence – 2008–09 Under-5 growth faltering: 16.1%	 2008–09: 2012: 2014:	Decreases in under-5 mortality CMR 84/1,000 CMR 73/1,000 CMR 52/1,000

*CMR = under-5 child mortality rate.

Table 1.2. Tanzania's History of Child Health, 1952–2016

[1] Macroeconomic, Political and Social Factors →	*[2] Community Conditions* →		*[3] Health Outcome*
PERIOD I (pre-1961) Colonial Era	– Poor water and sanitation – Impoverishment in monetized economy – Prenatal and postnatal care inadequate – Few rural health centers – Colonial violence + Liberation movement and community health	 1952: 1959: 1960: 1961:	Increases in under-5 mortality during colonial era, and slight decreases CMR* 206/1,000 CMR 220/1,000 CMR 219/1,000 CMR 218/1,000
	Period II Contextual Considerations ↓		
PERIOD II (1961–1996) Political independence and change in health policy	+ 1963 Zanzibar attains independence + 1967 Arusha Declaration – 1977 SAPs Instituted – 1978 Libya and Idi Amin attempt to annex Kagera, Tanzania's Northern Province + 1979 Tanzanian Army helps to oust Amin + 1994 Tanzania accepts 800,000 refugees from Rwanda and Burundi, straining community resources	 1971: 1981: 1991–92: 1996:	Lowered child mortality CMR 197/1,000 CMR 166/1,000 CMR 153/1,000 CMR 145/1,000

(continued)

Table 1.2. *(Continued)*

[1] Macroeconomic, Political and Social Factors	→	*[2] Community Conditions*	→	*[3] Health Outcome*
		Period III Contextual Consideration ↓		
PERIOD III (1996–99) Third decade of nationhood		+ Continued arrivals of refugees from Rwanda and Burundi	 1996: 1999:	Temporary increase in early childhood mortality (1996–99) CMR 145/1,000 CMR 161/1,000
		Period IV Contextual Considerations ↓		
PERIOD IV (1999–2016) Fourth and fifth decades of nationhood		+ 2000 East African Community Treaty – 2004–05 Under-5 stunting: 44% – 2010 Under-5 stunting: 42% + 2006 African Development Bank cancels >$640m of debt – 2014 Under-5 stunting: 35% +2016 Arrival of refugees from South Sudan	 2004–05: 2010: 2011: 2012:	Steady and impressive decreases in early childhood mortality CMR 132/1,000 CMR 92/1,000 CMR 81/1,000 CMR 54/1,000

*CMR = under-5 child mortality rate.

Table 1.3. Uganda's History of Child Health, 1953–2016

[1] Macroeconomic, Political and Social Factors	➔	*[2] Community Conditions*	➔	*[3] Health Outcome*
PERIOD I (pre-1962) Colonial Era		– Lack of schools – Uneven development infrastructure – Poor water and sanitation – Impoverishment in monetized economy – Prenatal and postnatal care inadequate – Few rural health centers – Colonial violence + Liberation movement and community health	 1953: 1961:	High child mortality CMR* 202/1,000 CMR 201/1,000
		Period II Contextual Considerations ⬇		
PERIOD II (1962–71) Political independence and change in health policy		+/– 1967 One-party state – 1971 Idi Amin overthrows Obote – Asians expelled from Uganda	 1962: 1965: 1971:	Lowered child mortality CMR 197/1,000 CMR 184/1,000 CMR 167/1,000

(continued)

Table 1.3. *(Continued)*

[1] Macroeconomic, Political and Social Factors	➔	*[2] Community Conditions*	➔	*[3] Health Outcome*
		Period III Contextual Consideration ➔		
PERIOD III (1972–87) Violence; several hundred thousand lose lives; political and economic destabilization		– Political and economic upheaval – Indiscriminate killings by Idi Amin – 1971–79: 300,000 Ugandans lose lives –/+ 1979 Amin overthrown – 1980–85 Obote II Regime: 300,000 Ugandans lose lives –/+ 1986 Museveni takes office as president; NRC bans political party activity in Uganda; Commission of Inquiry of Human Rights Violations established	1972: 1981: 1982: 1987:	*Increasing* child morbidity and mortality CMR 168/1,000 CMR 214/1,000 CMR 213/1,000 CMR 173/1,000
		Period IV Contextual Considerations ➔		
PERIOD IV (1988–2014) Debt relief, Poverty Eradication Program, National Water Policy		+ Ugandan troops help oust Mobutu – 2002 LRA attacks villages; Army relocates 400,000 – 2007 Floods and devastation –/+ 2010 Government corruption investigations – 2012 Aid halted by Britain and EU for theft – 2014 World Bank halts $90m; sanctions + "Some for all," not "all for some" + 2016 Refugees arriving from South Sudan	1988–89: 1995: 2000–01: 2006: 2011:	Initial decrease in under-5 mortality followed by stagnation (1995–2001) before 50-point decrease (2001–11) CMR 187/1,000 CMR 156/1,000 CMR 156/1,000 CMR 144/1,000 CMR 106/1,000

*CMR = under-5 child mortality rate.

Table 1.4. Kenya Milestones Relevant to Water, Sanitation, and Health

1940	Wangaari Maathai is born in Nyeri, Kenya.
1944	Kenya African Union is formed to campaign for independence.
1947	Jomo Kenyatta becomes leader of the Kenya African Union.
1963	Kenya gains independence from Britain. Jomo Kenyatta becomes prime minister.
1971	Wangari Maathai receives a Ph.D. from the University of Nairobi in veterinary anatomy, the first woman in East and Central Africa to earn a doctorate.
1972	Daniel Arap Moi becomes Kenya's second president.
1976	Professor Wangari Maathai begins planting trees (literally and figuratively).
1977	Professor Wangari Maathai founds the Green Belt Movement, which has planted 45 million trees in Kenya
1982	An attempted coup is suppressed by the army.
1991	The Forum for the Restoration of Democracy, led by J. Oginda Odinga, is formed.
1992	Multiparty elections are held; President Moi wins.
1997	Moi wins his second and final term as president.
2002	Raila Odinga and Mwai Kibaki form an opposition party/coalition that defeats Uhuru Kenyatta of Kenya African National Union.
2004	Professor Wangari Maathai is awarded the Nobel Peace Prize—the first to an African woman and the first "green Nobel."
2007	An elections dispute and turmoil transpire.
2011	East Africa is hit by the worst drought in 60 years.
2011	Dr. Wangari Maathai dies.
2012	Oil is discovered, hailed by President Kibaki as a "major breakthrough."
2013	Peaceful general elections and a landmark Supreme Court ruling uphold the presidential victory of Uhuru Kenyatta (son of Jomo Kenyatta).
2013	The British government says it sincerely regrets the torture of thousands of Kenyans during the suppression of the Mau Mau insurgency in the 1950s and promises £20m in compensation.
2014	Kenya is the fourth biggest economy in sub-Saharan Africa.

Table 1.5. Tanzania Milestones Relevant to Water, Sanitation, and Health

1905–07	The Maji Maji Revolt is suppressed by German troops.
1919–1961	British Indirect Rule (Africans of higher status became civil servants of British rule).
1929	The Tanganyika African Association is founded.
1954	Julius Nyerere and Oscar Kambona transform the Tanganyika African Association into the Tanganyika African National Union (TANU).
1961	Nyerere engineers independence for Tanganyika and becomes its first prime minister.
1964	Tanganyika joins Zanzibar to become the United Republic of Tanzania.
1967	Nyerere delivers the Arusha Declaration, calling for egalitarianism, socialism, and self-reliance.
1975	Rural villages project fails; farmers met their own needs and did not deliver on communal contributions.
1977	SAPs (Structural Adjustment Programs) are instituted, with a deleterious effect on women.
1979	Tanzania forces invade Uganda and help to oust President Idi Amin.
1985	Nyerere retires and is replaced by Ali Hassan Mwinyi.
1992	The constitution is amended to allow for multiparty democracy.
1995	Benjamin Mkapa is elected president.
1999	Julius Nyerere dies.
2000	Mkapa is elected for a second term with 72% of the vote.
2005	Jakaya Kikwete wins presidential elections, replacing Mkapa, who retires.
2006	Visiting Chinese prime minister Wen Jiabao signs an agreement to help Tanzania's health, transport and communications sectors.
2010	President Kikwete wins reelection.
2012	The Satoil and Exxon Mobil oil exploration companies make the biggest offshore discovery to date of gas reserves off the coast of Tanzania.
2013	Human Rights Watch reports that thousands of children work in small-scale Tanzania gold mines, at great risk to their health.
2015	John Magufuli, presenting the Chama Cha Mapinduzi Party, elected president.

Table 1.6. Uganda Milestones Relevant to Water, Sanitation, and Health

1962	Uganda gains independence from Britain; Dr. Milton Apollo Obote, leader of the Uganda People's Congress, becomes prime minister.
1963	Kabaka Mutesa II, king of Buganda, is elected ceremonial president of Uganda.
1966	The offices of prime minister and president are merged and Uganda is declared a republic.
1967	Obote abolished all monarchs, creating a one-party state.
1971	Idi Amin overthrows Obote; a campaign of terror is unleashed, and South Asians are expelled.
1971–79	During Amin's regime, 300,000 Ugandans lose their lives through indiscriminate extrajudicial killings.
1979	At the behest of the Uganda National Liberation Front (UNLF), the Uganda National Liberation Army (UNLA) and the Tanzania Peoples Defense Fund (TPDF) overthrow Amin's regime.
1980	General elections are held and Obote regains the presidency.
1980–85	300,000 Ugandans lose their lives and the economy is shattered.
1981	Yoweri Museveni leads the National Resistance Army (NRA) to engage in a war of liberation.
1985	The UNLA (but not NRA) ousts Obote; the military junta of generals Bazillo and Tito Okello replaces Obote.
1986	The Okellos' junta is ousted by the National Resistance Army (NRA), "an uprising of oppressed Ugandan citizens" (Uganda High Commission, Ottawa, Canada).
1986	Yoweri Museveni is sworn in as president of the Republic of Uganda.
1995	A new constitution creates a nonparty, all-inclusive "movement system" of government.
1998	Uganda troops help depose Zaire's military dictator and president Mobutu Sese Seko, who is replaced by Laurent Kabila.
2001	The East African Community (EAC)—its members being Tanzania, Uganda, and Kenya—is inaugurated in Arusha, laying the groundwork for a common East African passport and flag and economic and monetary integration.
2001	Museveni is reelected as Uganda's president, winning 69% of the vote.
2002	A Ugandan rebel group, the Lord's Resistance Army (LRA), brutally attacks villages. The army evacuates 400,000 civilians.
2005	July: A national referendum resolves to return to multiparty politics. October: An international criminal court issues arrest warrants for five LRA commanders, including leader Joseph Kony. December: The international court in The Hague rules that Uganda must compensate the Democratic Republic of the Congo for rights abuses and plundering of resources in the five years leading to 2003.
2006	Multiparty elections are held, with President Yoweri Museveni winning 59% of the vote and the National Resistance movement winning the highest number of seats in Parliament.
2007	September: A state of emergency is imposed after severe floods cause widespread devastation.

(continued)

Table 1.6. ***(Continued)***

2008	November: LRA leader Joseph Kony again fails to turn up for the signing of a peace agreement. Armies from Uganda, South Sudan, and the Democratic Republic of the Congo launch an offensive against LRA bases.
2009	January: The LRA appeals for a ceasefire in the face of a continuing offensive by regional countries. UK oil explorer Heritage Oil claims a major oil find in Uganda. December: Parliament votes to ban female circumcision, with anyone convicted of the practice to face 10 years in jail or a life sentence if a victim dies.
2010	January: President Museveni distances himself from the antihomosexuality bill, saying the ruling party MP who proposed the bill did so as an individual. The European Union and United States had condemned the bill.
2010	February: Heritage Oil sells its assets in Uganda to UK firm Tullow Oil after Italian energy company Eni drops out of the bidding.
2010	June: Public prosecutor opens corruption investigation against Vice-President Gilbert Bukenya, Foreign Minister Sam Kutesa and several other ministers and officials over the alleged theft of $25m.
2010	October: The UN report into killing of Hutus in Democratic Republic of the Congo between 1993 and 2003 says they may constitute "crimes of genocide." It implicates Rwanda, Uganda, Burundi, Zimbabwe, and Angola.
2011	February: Museveni wins his fourth presidential election. Challenger Kizza Besigye alleges vote-rigging and dismisses the result as a sham.
2011	July: The United States deploys Special Forces personnel to help Uganda combat LRA rebels.
2012	May: The Ugandan army captures senior LRA commander Caesar Achellam in a clash in the Central African Republic, one of the nearby states in which the remaining band of LRA troops operates. Billing Achellam as a top LRA strategist, Uganda says this is a major breakthrough. Tens of thousands of refugees cross into Uganda, fleeing fighting in the Democratic Republic of the Congo.
2012	November: Uganda announces its intention to withdraw from UN-backed international peacekeeping missions in response to UN accusations that Uganda is arming Congolese rebels. Britain and other European countries halt aid channeled through the Ugandan government amid a scandal involving the alleged theft of donor funds.
2013	March: At a meeting of CITES, the body regulating wildlife trade, Uganda is grouped among the worst offenders in the illegal ivory trade.
2013	May: The government temporarily shuts down two newspapers after they publish a letter suggesting President Museveni is grooming his son for power.
2013	December: Parliament passes a controversial antigay bill that increases the punishments for homosexual acts, to include life imprisonment.
2014	February: President Museveni signs the tough new antigay bill into law, drawing criticism from around the world. The World Bank postpones a $90m (£54m) loan to Uganda over the move, and the United States imposes sanctions.

In Kenya, estimates of under-5 mortality rates before colonialism vary widely, from as high as 383 deaths per 1,000 live births in 1950 to a low rate of 169 deaths per 1,000 live births in 1963, at independence, according to estimates generated by the United Nations Inter-agency Group for Child Mortality Estimation (IGME) in 2014. Uneven development of the country typifies Period I (see Table 1.1, column 1, first panel). Colonial violence led to the disenfranchisement of African populations in Kenya. Settlers moved to the highlands and created development infrastructure, such as the railroad from Mombasa to Lake Victoria, for their own interests. Kenyans fought multiple wars of liberation. The Kenyan African Union was eventually victorious, and Jomo Kenyatta became the first prime minister of the newly liberated territory. Women's roles are recognized in Kenya, exemplified by Wangari Maathai, born during colonial rule in 1940, being the first woman in East Africa to earn a doctoral degree, in 1971 (see Table 1.4).

During Period II (Table 1.1, second panel), the first 25 years of Kenya's postcolonial history, early childhood survival improved, from 164 deaths per 1,000 live births to 91. However, Ngare and Muttunga (1999) report an upward trend in under-5 growth faltering during this period. Wangari Maathai founded the Green Belt movement and was responsible for planting 45 *million* trees. Political upheaval was present during this period, as the military thwarted a 1982 coup attempt and in 1987 opposition groups were suppressed and the government was criticized internationally for human rights abuses.

In Period III (Table 1.1, third panel), corruption, ethnic tensions, and rent battles abounded. Due to corruption, the World Bank withheld $5 billion in structural adjustment credit. In an important influx of funds, Maasai and Samburu groups accepted $7 million from the British government for its human rights abuses during Kenya's wars for liberation, leading to death and maiming of countless individuals. However, much of the country endured economic hardship as the IMF suspended lending to Kenya in 2000 for three years. While child morbidity varied during this period, child survival took a hit. Under-5 mortality per 1,000 live births rose to 93 deaths in 1993 and further to 115 in 2003. In 2003 15.8% of Kenyan children under the age of 5 were experiencing chronic malnutrition, leading to growth faltering.

In the fourth and final period under examination (Table 1.1, fourth panel), under-5 mortality in Kenya decreased and early childhood morbidity increased. Corruption was still rampant among government officials, and citizens experienced multiple province-wide food crises. Kenyans protested for land and water rights, and 35,000 refugees entered the country from Somalia. Election violence also ensued in 2006 and 2008.

A report on "changes in child mortality in a rural area of Kenya during 2003–2009, when major public health interventions were scaled-up" (Hamel et al. 2011) found that

> [m]ortality remained elevated during the first 8 months of 2009 compared with 2006 and 2007. Malaria and/or anemia accounted for the greatest increases in child mortality. Stock-outs of essential antimalarial drugs during a time of increased malaria transmission and disruption of services during civil unrest may have contributed to increased mortality in 2008–2009. (p. 597)

Consistent with findings from Hamel et al. (2011), growth faltering among children under the age of five increased to 16.1%, but despite Kenya's political and economic challenges, the country's under-5 mortality rate decreased to 84 deaths per 1,000 live births in 2008–09, according to the Kenya Demographic and Health Survey, and to 73 deaths per 1,000 live births in 2012, according to the UN.

In Tanzania, under-5 mortality increased in the 10 years preceding independence, according to the United Nations Inter-agency Group for Child Mortality Estimation (2014). In Period 1 (Table 1.2, first panel), the under-5 mortality rate rose from 206 deaths per 1,000 live births in 1952 to 220 deaths by 1959. Even in 1961 it lowered very slightly, to 218. In 1961, at the dawn of Period II, Julius Nyerere became the first prime minister of Tanganyika (see Table 1.5). Shortly thereafter Zanzibar attained independence, and in 1964 the two became the United Republic of Tanzania. In 1967 Nyerere issued the Arusha Declaration, calling for *Ujamaa* socialism. Though the country faced structural adjustment policies, an attempt by Libya and Idi Amin of Uganda to annex Kagera (one of Tanzania's Northern Provinces), and an influx of 800,000 refugees from Rwanda and Burundi, child survival improved. By 1996, under-5 mortality had decreased to 145 deaths per 1,000 live births.

Outside of the colonial period, Tanzania boasts a relatively prolonged and consistent drop in deaths among children under 5 compared with Kenya. However, the exception occurs in Period III, which I have marked off in my framework as a distinctive period, despite its very short length. In Period III (Table 1.2, third panel), under-5 mortality temporarily increased from 145 deaths per 1,000 live births in 1996 to 161 deaths in 1999, according to the Tanzania Demographic and Health Survey (National Bureau of Statistics/ Tanzania and Macro International 2000). In April 1994, 170,000 refugees from Rwanda arrived in Tanzania within 48 hours (Whitaker 2002). After a total of 600,000 had arrived, Tanzania closed it western border in March 1995. The border was reopened in January 1996, but by December 1996, "the Tanzanian government and the Office of the United Nations High Commissioner for Refugees (UNHCR) issued a joint statement that read, in part, 'all

Rwandese refugees in Tanzania are expected to return home by 31 December 1996'" (Whitaker 2002, 1). In examining data comparing infant and child mortality rates for 1991–1992, well before the refugees came from Rwanda, with rates from 1996, after the height of arrivals of Rwandans and before the deadline for their departure from Tanzania, certain regions appear to be more negatively affected by the impact of refugees, who at times outnumbered Tanzanian citizens in some communities. According to UNHCR (1997, 1),

> The highest refugee concentrations are in some of the poorest countries in the world. A large number of such movements are into least developed countries. The presence of refugees compounds the already prevailing economic, environmental, social and, at times, political difficulties in these countries. Often such countries are confronted by a combination of all four of these factors. Nearly always their impact is substantial. Moreover, in many refugee situations, problems are aggravated when refugees are a substantial proportion of the local, if not national population. For example, in Ngara, . . . in the United Republic of Tanzania, the recent refugee influxes meant that the local population was outnumbered by a ratio of approximately 4:1; i.e., there were some 700,000 refugees among a local population of 186,000. . . . The presence of refugees, and demands on the already severely strained economy, services and infrastructure add to the extreme hardship affecting the local populations. In many instances, refugees become an added impediment to, or risk jeopardizing, the development efforts of the host country. Their negative aspects may be felt long after a refugee problem is solved; for example, the damage to environment is a process and does not end with the repatriation of refugees.

The regions in which initial drops in infant and child mortality reversed in Tanzania, possibly as a result of the influx of refugees and other factors, include Northern, Southern, and Southern Highlands.

The regions with higher mortality rates for infants and/or children correspond more directly with those with high seropositive HIV rates among women. While regional data is not available for 1996 or 1999, extrapolating from 2010 regional data shows the Southern Highlands having the highest HIV rates and the largest differentials in infant and child mortality rates between 1992 and 1996. Mtwara, followed by Ruvuma in the Southern region, has the highest percentage of women who are seropositive, corresponding with the regions in 1996 DHS data that have worse child survival than in 1991–92. And Kilimanjaro, Tanga, followed by Arusha, has the highest HIV rates in the Northern region, corresponding with its higher infant and child mortality rates in 1996 compared with 1991–1992. Finally, Zanzibar's rates are not higher in 1996, but its infant and child mortality rates are higher in 1999 than in 1996, and the totals for the whole country of Tanzania are higher in 1999 than in 1996. And Zanzibar's HIV rates are among the highest in Tanzania. According to the U.S. Census Bureau, HIV seroprevalence for pregnant women in Dar es Salaam reached its peak in 1999 at 16%.

In Period IV (Table 1.2, fourth panel), child mortality rates drop impressively from 132 deaths per 1,000 live births in 2004–2005 to 54 in 2012—less than half the 2004 rate. Tanzania was the only country in East Africa to meet Millennium Development Goals. In 2006, visiting Chinese prime minister Wen Jiabao signed an agreement to invest in Tanzania's health, transport, and communications sectors. And multinational corporate interests discovered gas reserves off the coast of Tanzania. It remains to be seen whether these investments and discoveries will ultimately benefit ordinary citizens of Tanzania. A case in point is that Human Rights Watch reports (2010) that thousands of children work in small-scale gold mines in the country.

In Uganda (Table 1.3, column 1, first panel), the colonial era occurred before 1962. Community conditions varied by region under colonial exploitation. For example, "the northern region was not developed during the colonial period, and served mainly as a reservoir for cheap labor to be deployed in the south"; and "Britain recruited its soldiers mostly from the northern region" (Bouckaert 1999). These North–South tensions, exacerbated by a divide-and-rule strategy imposed by the British, still factor in Uganda's internal disputes today.

As shown in the timeline in Table 1.6, Uganda gained independence in 1962. In the period from 1953 to 1961, the under-5 mortality rate fell slightly from 2002 to 2001. In Period II, the first decade of independence, Uganda became a one-party state. In 1971, Idi Amin overthrew President Obote and expelled South Asians from the country. Despite these violent political contests, the under-5 mortality rate fell from 197 deaths per 1,000 live births in 1962 to 167 deaths in 1971.

In Period III, nearing the close of the first decade of independence, Idi Amin's coup instigated *increasing* under-5 mortality rates from 1971 until 1981. Under-5 mortality increased by 45 points to a high of 214 deaths for every 1,000 born—more than one in five children dying before a fifth birthday. In addition to hunger and disease, injury accounts for numerous deaths, as 300,000 lost their lives during the years of violence wrought against Uganda's citizens.

> In any contemporary lexicon of horror, Uganda is synonymous with state-become-slaughterhouse. The most conservative estimates by informed observers hold that President Idi Amin Dada and the terror squads operating under his loose direction have killed 100,000 Ugandans in the seven years he has held power. Some estimates run as high as 300,000. Many victims have been guilty

> of nothing more than catching the eye of the killer—a shopkeeper with coveted goods, a Christian in a Muslim village, a civil servant who questions a command, a judge with foreign friends. (Ullman 1978, p. 529)

Amin and his forces engaged in a "clean-up" campaign "to establish Amin's authority as a leader and provide the state with a more 'legitimate' means of eliminating political dissent" (Decker 2010, p. 491). Unfortunately, the killings did not stop with the overthrow of Amin in 1979. From 1980 to 1985, "under Obote, state-sanctioned murder and the uncontrolled army predations continued." (Reid 2014, p. 374)

> By 1984, the U.S. State Department estimated that between 100,000 and 200,000 civilians were slaughtered in the Luwero triangle by the Obote regime, and by 1985, the number was believed to be far higher. . . . After the war ended in 1986, the International Committee of the Red Cross claimed that at least 300,000 people had died in the Luwero triangle and that officials had failed to account for half to a third of the region's population. (Bouckaert 1999)

Loss of life and livelihood and "heavy devaluation of the Ugandan shilling" (Mutibwa 1992) led to a downward spiral in Uganda's economy. From 1980 to 1985, the average income per head of population fell by nearly 2% each year, "and "inflation was rising even faster" (Mutibwa 1992, p. 152). In 1986, after contestation with groups fighting to oust Obote, Museveni and his National Resistance Movements took power and he was established as president. The National Resistance Council was established, and Museveni banned political activity and created a Commission of Inquiry of Human Rights Violations (Human Rights Watch 2010).

In the final period (Period IV) noted in Table 1.3, an initial increase in under-5 mortality to 187 deaths per 1,000 live births was followed by a decrease to 156 deaths in the 1995 and 2000–2001 DHS. Thereafter under-5 mortality decreased to 106 deaths in 2011, a 108-point drop from 1982 rates. Though rates of child survival were improving, political and economic volatility and military interventions continued as Ugandan troops fought to oust Mobutu in the Congo, The Lord's Resistance Army fought in the North, and government officials' corruption withdrew needed resources from ordinary citizens. Continued human rights violations and corruptions eroded international aid efforts and forestalled World Bank investments.

In the current epoch, refugee support has impacted community resources in Uganda. In 2015, Uganda was host to the eighth largest number of refugees worldwide. And with many new arrivals from South Sudan, from 2015 to 2016 there was a 68% increase in the number of refugees in Uganda. The total there in 2016 was 1,162,715 (UNHCR 2017).

> The total number of South Sudanese refugees has now passed 1.4 million; it is the largest refugee crisis in Africa, and the third largest in the world, after Syria and Afghanistan. There are nearly two million people who have been forced to flee their homes but remain in South Sudan and another 250,000 refugees in South Sudan from neighboring countries.[2]

Uganda is a host country to refugees principally from South Sudan and the Congo, though some Rwandan refugees remain. According to Zerai, Olemako, Morrow, and Guest (2017, 5):

> UNHCR relies on voluntary contributions from governments and the private sector, making funding limited and placing the financial burden on host communities that may be unable to accommodate and safeguard large influxes of displaced persons.[3] In Uganda, these resource challenges are extensive, but the country has come to be considered one of the most favorable refugee environments in the world.[4] Uganda's refugee population is at one of the highest points in its history. . . . The country currently hosts a disproportionately high number of women and children (for example, 86% of South Sudanese refugees in the country are women and children), and holistic solutions are required to meet the needs of these vulnerable populations.[5]

For an already overtaxed infrastructure, the country of Uganda not only continues to find ways to support its neighbors in crisis, but it is also making strides in its efforts to equitably distribute resources to its citizenry.

"Some for All" versus "All for Some"

In 1998 Uganda implemented water sector reforms. After receiving widespread input from citizens, values guiding the reforms were agreed to, including a focus on poverty reduction, and determining a sector-wide approach to water and sanitation. A hallmark of these changes was that donors' agendas no longer determined water investments. Water sector plans were made and donor inputs were only accepted to the extent that they supported the sectorwide strategic planning efforts. This meant that Uganda's National Water Policy could determine "resource allocation . . . on the principle of 'some for all' rather than 'all for some.' The policy also stipulates that interventions should respond to differing needs, and specifically highlights the central role of women in sanitation. Men and women's equal opportunity to participate in all aspects of community development is considered a guiding principle for the focus of activities in the sector" (WHO 2015, p. 18). The World Health Organization has lauded these aspects of Uganda's National Water Policy.

A "DAY IN THE LIVES" OF WOMEN AND GIRLS IN KENYA, TANZANIA, AND UGANDA

As noted previously, the exigent realities of coups, the displacement of hundreds of thousands of people—due to political upheaval, war, unpredictable climate change, and myriad other circumstances—have measurable effects on the lives of women and girls in East Africa. Hunger is not the same everywhere. For example, as late as 1982 in Uganda, 213 children out of 1,000 born were dying before the age of 5. That means that in a family of 7 siblings (Uganda's total fertility rate in 1982 was 7.1 births per woman), an average of one or two were dying per family—losing a sibling was commonplace due to diarrhea or diarrheal diseases, malaria, pneumonia, or injuries from war. These of course were not equal opportunity losses of the lives of loved ones. While some siblings may have remained alive in some families, other children lost numerous brothers and/or sisters. In this section, I aim describe how the lives of women and children are shaped by their contexts.

Women and Children in Kenya, 2014

A sociological imagination helps us to understand the intersection of biography and history in the lives of girls in Kenya. Drilling down to data elucidates the context. According the DHS, for example, there has been an increase in the percentage of girls attending primary school, both in urban and rural areas of Kenya. And, if we take a look at the most recent Kenya DHS, we see that net attendance ratio in primary education among 6-13 year-olds is 85.5 out of 100 among males and 87.6 out of 100 among females. However, there is wide variation by region, where in the North Eastern region, for example, only 51% of girls and 60% of boys ages 6-13 are attending primary school (Kenya National Bureau of Statistics [KNBS] and ICF 2015). In children's own words, we see the demand for school attendance. In the poem showcased at Girls Speak Out, United Nations Day of the Girl, October 2014, "What It Means to Be a Girl in My Village," Koipano Kimeker and Felistus Gilai, 4th graders at the Kakenya Center for Excellence, remark, *"you may think I went to school, but I didn't; the reason is because I am a girl."* They admonish, *"Parents take your children to school, for one day they will help you remember education is the key to life"* (Kimeker and Gilai 2014).

Rapid Urbanization and Development Infrastructure

There is rapid urbanization in Kenya. In 2010, 76% of women lived in rural areas of Kenya, and by 2014, that number dropped to 59% (Kenya National

Bureau of Statistics [KNBS] and ICF Macro 2010), and this number dropped to 33% by 2014. The majority of women are literate (88% according to the Kenya National Bureau of Statistics [KNBS] and ICF 2015). Currently, 36% have electricity in their homes, ranging from 68% in urban areas to 13% in rural areas. Regarding water and sanitation, 71% of households obtain drinking water from improved sources, with the number at 59% in rural areas. Improved toilet facilities are less available. Unshared flush toilets are available to only 8% of households (1% in rural areas, 17% in urban areas). A lack of electricity means that that 59% of Kenyan households use wood, straw, shrubs, and grass for cooking fuel, with deleterious effects on women's health and the environment. Wood is used in 84% of rural areas and 17% of urban areas. In urban areas, charcoal (28%) and kerosene (27%) are used most frequently (2014 data from Kenya National Bureau of Statistics [KNBS] and ICF 2015).

Water for drinking was found on site for 28% of all women of childbearing age in Kenya in 2014 (Kenya National Bureau of Statistics [KNBS] and ICF 2015, analyzed data). In urban households, a majority of women either had water on site (54%) or walked less than 30 minutes to obtain it (33%), whereas in rural areas the majority of women who lacked water on premises walked 30 minutes or longer to obtain it (40%). Only 27% of rural households had drinking water on the premises; females over 15 constituted the majority who collected drinking water. In urban areas, half (47%) treated drinking water; about half either boiled their water or used bleach/chorine to treat it. In rural areas, 45% of households used an appropriate method to treat drinking water.

Women's Employment, Marital Status, and Empowerment

At this same time, women who were employed were in better circumstances relative to women in Uganda and Tanzania. Sixty-one percent of women were employed in the past year. They worked in professional, technical, or managerial occupations (14%), or in sales and services (14%); 31% were in agriculture, and 28% were in domestic service. In Kenya in 2014 66% were paid in cash only, 18% were not paid, and 17% received earnings with in-kind or a mix of in-kind and cash payments (Kenya National Bureau of Statistics [KNBS] and ICF 2015). Of employed women, only 12% earned more than their partners, and only 10% of employed women did not decide how to spend their earnings (analyzed data.)

In terms of women's empowerment, in 2014 (Kenya National Bureau of Statistics [KNBS] and ICF 2015) men had higher educational attainment, but women's levels of education were still higher in Kenya than in Uganda and Tanzania; 67% of women and 72% of men completed primary or more education, and 27% of women and 33% of men completed higher education and/or secondary school. The gender gap has narrowed but continues to be present with completed secondary and postsecondary educational attainment.

Most marriages (90% in urban areas and 84% in rural areas) among women ages 15 to 49 were monogamous. The North Eastern province has the most polygynous marriages (32%). Most women ages 20–24 are married (55%). Men marry on average 5 years later; only 18% are married by between the ages of 20–24%, and 57% are married between ages of 25–29 (Kenya National Bureau of Statistics [KNBS] and ICF 2015). Women's husbands are generally 5 years older (as shown by differences in median age at first marriage; Kenya Demographic and Health Survey 2014). Women's median age at first sexual intercourse is 18; men's is age 17. The total fertility rate is 3.9 births per woman (3.1 in urban areas and 4.5 in rural areas).

HIV prevalence among adults in Kenya has declined from 10% in the 1990s to 5.4% in 2016, and HIV prevalence among males is 5.6%, and 7.6% among women (UNAIDS 2017). A previous survey shows rates range from as low as .8% among those of Somali ethnicity to a high of 20.2% among Luo peoples (Kenya National Bureau of Statistics [KNBS] and ICF Macro 2010).

By and large, husbands and wives work together to make decisions about health care, major household purchases, daily household needs, and wives' travel. Even with major household purchases, husbands and wives determine these jointly in 73% of households among currently married women (Kenya National Bureau of Statistics [KNBS] and ICF 2015). Kenya by and large appears to have higher levels of gender equity than Tanzania and Uganda. However, the North Eastern province is the outlier in this regard; there 63% of married women make decisions about their own health care (compared with 79% of married women in all provinces).

A significant proportion of women (42%) and over one-third of men (36%) agree with wife beating, or physical abuse, under a number of circumstances, including neglect of children. Some women (15%) and 10% of men agree that wife beating is justified if a woman refuses to have sex with her husband. And 21% of women and 2% of men agree that it is justified is a wife argues with her husband (Kenya National Bureau of Statistics [KNBS] and ICF 2015). These percentages are highest among men in the North Eastern province (Kenya National Bureau of Statistics [KNBS] and ICF 2015).

Physical violence against women is still widespread in Kenya: 45% of women ages 15 to 49 have experienced physical violence after the age of 15 (Kenya National Bureau of Statistics [KNBS] and ICF Macro 2015). A majority of women who live in the Nyanza region (57%), Nairobi (54%), and

Western region (53%) have experienced physical violence after the age of 15. Of all married women who had been assaulted, 57% were assaulted by their current husbands. Of never-married women, 48% were assaulted by teachers, 40% by mothers or stepmothers, and 19% by fathers or stepfathers. Twenty-two percent of women who have experienced sexual violence live in Nyanza; and 22% live in Western province. Fourteen percent of women ages 15 to 49 have ever experienced sexual violence in Kenya. Perpetrators have been current husband/partners and current or former boyfriends among never-married women. Beyond their partners, never-married women were sexually assaulted by friends/acquaintances and by strangers.

Women and Children in Tanzania, 2015–2016

According to the DHS data from Tanzania, collected in 2015–2016, 85% of urban females ages 15–49 have completed primary education or more. In urban areas, 39% have completed some secondary education or more. The picture in rural areas has improved from previous surveys; 67% of women have completed primary education or more, and 15% have gone on to secondary education. Gender equity in education seems to be better achieved in Tanzania relative to Kenya and Uganda. Of males ages 15–49, 87% have completed primary-level or more education in urban areas and 70% in rural areas. With regards to median years of education, gender equity exists at 6.5 median years *for both men and women* 15–49. Impressively, across the board (considering rural/urban residence, region, wealth, etc.), gender parity indexes (GPIs) for Tanzania range from .94 (favoring males) to 1.19 (favoring females), with a GPI for the country overall of 1.08. This is the most equitable rate for primary school attendance in East Africa. The rural rate is higher in Tanzania (GPI 1.09) than in Kenya and Uganda (Tanzania Central Statistical Office and Institute for Resource Development/Macro Systems 2016; Kenya National Bureau of Statistics [KNBS] and ICF Macro 2015; Uganda Bureau of Statistics [UBOS] and Institute for Resource Development/Macro Systems 2011). The literacy rate for women—76%—is high in Tanzania, but only 49% in the lowest-wealth quintile are literate. For men, 77% are literate, and 55% in the lowest-wealth quintile. This indicates some gender disparity among the poor.

Water and Sanitation in Tanzania

Drinking water from improved sources (such as piped into dwelling, shared tap, public tap, tube well, protected dug well, protected spring or rainwater) is more available across the board in Tanzania than in Kenya and Uganda. Over half of women's households (61%) have access to improved sources. In urban areas access to improved sources of drinking water is higher (86%)

than in rural areas (49%); and Zanzibar has almost universal access to improved sources (98%). A small proportion of households have access to water in their residence or yard/plot (or both)—25% in urban areas, 4% in rural areas, and 37% in Zanzibar. Women walk less than 30 minutes on average to obtain water. About a third (30%) of households boil water prior to drinking it; 61% do not treat their drinking water. Contaminated water is still a cause of disease, as only 33% of drinking water consumed is judged to be treated appropriately (Tanzania Central Statistical Office and Institute for Resource Development/Macro Systems [from here referred to as "TDHS," for "Tanzania Demographic and Health Survey"] 2016).

Improved toilet facilities are in short supply in Tanzania; only 19% access improved facilities, including flush toilets, ventilated improved pit latrines, or pit latrines with slab that are not shared by members of more than one household. Similar to the rest of the continent, only 23% of households have electricity. Cooking fuel tends to be wood (6% of households), followed by charcoal (27%).

Employment, Fertility, Marriage and Violence

In the 12 months before the 2016 TDHS survey, 72% of women (and 88% of men) were employed, but this percentage includes young persons ages 15 to 19 who may have been in school. Women in urban areas were almost twice as likely to be employed than those in rural areas. This together with education and literacy averages bodes well for women's empowerment in rural areas. Most women (56%) work in the agricultural sector; 22% work in unskilled manual occupations. Almost half of women (53%) received cash for their earnings; 38% are not paid.

Total fertility rates are similar to those in many African countries: 3.8 in urban areas (which is slightly higher than some countries) and 6.0 in rural areas (which is similar). Given that more women in urban areas do not have employment, it appears that a traditional domesticity is upheld in many households in Tanzania. Median birth interval is relatively lengthy, at 35 months (TDHS 2016). Most women wait until they are 20 to give birth to their first child.

Median age at first marriage is 19.2 for women and 24.3 for men (TDHS 2016). Co-wives are relatively rare in Tanzania; 18% of ever-married women have co-wives, and 91.5% of ever-married men are married to only one wife. These factors have a positive association with women's empowerment in Tanzania.

As in other countries, women's first "sexual encounters" are reported to happen earlier than men's; median age at first sexual "intercourse for men 25–49 is 18.2 years. Whereas the median age for women . . . is 17.2 years"

(TDHS 2016: 85). More women ages 20 to 49 (13.2%) reported having first intercourse by the age of 15, compared with 9.6% for men. Some reports read that "men tend to initiate sexual activity later in life than women" (TDHS 2016), but these statistics reveal that the earlier sexual encounters are due to earlier marriage and betrothal to older men and to sexual assault of teen girls by older men. Though not available in TDHS 2015–2016, in 2011 data, in fact, among sexually active women, 11.3% were raped (captured in TDHS 2011 as "forced at sexual initiation") before the age of 15, and 10.5% were raped from ages 15 to 19. At ages 20 to 24, 9% were raped, and at ages 25 to 29, 4.5% were raped (prior to their first consensual sexual encounter, TDHS 2011). It is troubling that the TDHS 2011 reports this as a sexual encounter and not as violence.

Access to health care is problematic for many, but these problems are less widespread in Tanzania than in Kenya and Uganda. The highest percentages of women who have trouble accessing health care are those who live in the Southern zone, who have no education, who are in the lowest-wealth quintile, who are employed but are not paid in cash, and who have 5 or more children. Overall, 66% of women in Tanzania have at least one problem accessing health care.

Only 17% of women's husbands decide how to spend women's cash earnings, and 73% of husbands earned more than their wives in 2016. Decisions about major household purchases were made mainly by husbands (64%, decisions about purchases). Even in terms of a woman's own health care, mainly husbands decide for 28% of married women. This is especially egregious in the Central zone and Southern Highlands where 80.4% and 83.2% of husbands, respectively, decide on wives' own health care, and in Dodoma, Kilimanjaro, Morogoro, Dar es Salaam, Ruvuma, Simiyu, Njombe, Kaskazini Pemba, and Kusini Pemba, where over 79% make these decisions for their wives. Much to my surprise, women whose households are in the highest-wealth quintile and who have the highest educational levels also have the highest percentages of husbands who make health care decisions on their behalf: 82% of women with secondary or more education compared with 61% with no education, and 80% of women in the highest-wealth quintile compared with 64% of the lowest. Wife beating is all too common, and over half of women (58%) agree that women should be beaten under certain conditions. For example, 42% of women believe a wife should be beaten if she argues with her husband.

Past the age of 15, 44% of women have ever experienced physical violence (including sexual violence), as reported in TDHS 2015–2016. Of those experiencing violence past the age of 15, 48% of ever-married abused women experienced the violence at the hands of their current husband and/or partner and 40% from a former husband and/or partner. Of never-married women, 42% experienced violence from their current/former boyfriend; a "friend" or acquaintance assaulted 31%.

Women and Children in Uganda, 2011

Women in Uganda have very different experiences according to residence (especially those living in Kampala compared with the rest of the country), marital status, education, wealth, age, and ability. Their life choices as girls are much affected by their access to secondary education. According to Demographic and Health Survey data collected in 2011, female literacy rates are generally lower than male literacy rates, and vary widely by region, from 22% in Karamoja to 91% in Kampala. And only 20% of women in rural regions have attended secondary school, whereas in urban regions the rate is 58.9%. And higher percentages of men attended secondary school relative to women, regardless of the type of place of residence. While primary school attendance rates in 2011 were close to parity (GPIs of 1.03 in urban areas, .95 in rural areas), secondary school attendance is .93 in urban areas and a shocking .66 in rural areas, both favoring male children. In Kampala, Uganda's capital city, the gender parity index is .57, tied with the North region as the lowest GPI. A GPI lower than 1 indicates a gender disparity in favor of males (Uganda Bureau of Statistics [UBOS] and Institute for Resource Development/Macro Systems 2011).

Coupled with these educational inequities are gender gaps in entry into first marriage, first sexual intercourse, and childbearing. Young women are partnered with older men in each of these experiences, affecting their power within their households. Further, 26% of women in rural areas and 20% of women living in urban areas are co-wives in polygynous unions. High total fertility rates in Uganda of 4 children in urban areas and 7 in rural areas (which are the highest rates in eastern and southern Africa [Uganda Bureau of Statistics [UBOS] and Institute for Resource Development/Macro Systems 2011]) indicate highly defined traditionally gendered roles for women.

So what is a day like in the lives of women in Uganda? Consider the morning: Most women (80%) live in rural settings, where only 6% have water on their premises. Because women are primarily responsible for obtaining water for their households, they must get up early and walk to get the day's drinking water if it was not obtained the day before. In rural areas, almost a third of those walking for water (31%) travel less than 30 minutes, but the overwhelming majority (62%) travel more than 30 minutes. This means that over half of women throughout Uganda (54%) travel 30 minutes or longer each day to obtain drinking water for their households (Uganda Bureau of Statistics [UBOS] and Institute for Resource Development/Macro Systems 2011). Once water is obtained, it is boiled by 71% of urban households and 38% of rural households before drinking. In rural areas, 59% of households do not treat their drinking water, while a total of 53% do throughout the country.

Clean water is not plentiful, nor is electricity. In urban areas, 55% of residents have access to electricity in their homes, but only 5% in rural areas have access, so countrywide, only 15% have access to electricity. Sanitation needs are woefully inadequate. In rural areas, 73% of households use a pit latrine without a slab or an open pit, and 62% use the bush or fields to defecate. While some in urban areas have access to improved facilities, 52% of households utilize shared facilities. Flush toilets are available to only 9% of all households.

In obtaining water, cooking meals, and planning the day, it is important for women to consider who is in their household. The average household size is about 5 people, though it ranges as low as almost 4 in urban areas. Men head 71% of households. A third of households include foster and/or orphan children. Sleeping quarters are tight, as most households only have one room for sleeping (46% overall). Sleeping rooms are scarce in urban areas, where real estate costs more. In urban areas, households on average (62%) have one room for sleeping.

A Glimpse into Midday

In the 12 months before Uganda's 2011 DHS survey, 64% of women living in urban settings in Uganda and 70.5% in rural settings were employed. Most women work in skilled agriculture, forestry, and fishery work (57% of all women ages 15 to 49). In rural areas 67% of women were involved in these occupations, whereas in urban settings the majority of women worked in sales and service occupations (41%). For example, women in Kampala worked either in sales and services (46%) or in elementary occupations (e.g., "cleaners and helpers" according to Uganda Bureau of Statistics [UBOS] and Institute for Resource Development/Macro Systems 2011; 28%). Earnings type, another important indicator of power in the household, was largely cash and in-kind payments (24%) or in-kind payments only (5%) for women involved in agricultural work, except for the 36% of women who indicate that they were *not paid* for their agricultural work. This is 26% of all women ages 15 to 49 in Uganda, meaning that the majority of working women (51%) are either not paid at all or not paid a full wage.

Considerations for the Evening Hours

Domestic violence modules provide details on women's experiences in their marital households. Of ever-married women ages 15 to 49, 43% indicate they have experienced emotional violence from their spouses; 51% indicate they have experienced physical or sexual violence. Physical, sexual, or emotional violence is more likely to occur among women who are ages 20 or higher, who are Pentecostal, or who are Itesa (74%) or Banyankole (59%) ethnicity (though even 49% of Baganda women experience violence). Also, 61% of women in rural settings and 53% in urban settings report violence from their husband/partner. Women who have more children are more likely to experience violence (65.5% with 5 or more children compared with 44% of women with no children). And even 48% of women in the highest-wealth quintile have experienced partner violence. Marital control behaviors appear to predict violence against women: 74% of men displaying 5 or 6 controlling behaviors (such as tracking, jealousy, making accusations, and limiting interactions with others, including female friends and family members), and 26% of men displaying no controlling behaviors (in addition to violence) have physically assaulted their wives/partners[6] (Uganda Bureau of Statistics [UBOS] and Institute for Resource Development/Macro Systems 2011).

What Happens When Illness Strikes?

Women in Uganda report impediments to accessing health care, including getting permission from spouses to go for treatment (6% overall), getting money for treatment (49% overall), transportation problems that include distance to health facilities (41%), and feeling that they do not want to go alone for treatment (22%). Distance, for example, is a problem for half of women (48%) in rural areas and 13% in urban areas. Getting money for treatment is a problem for over half of women in rural households (53%) and 33% of urban households. Overall, 71% of women in rural settings and 40% in urban settings—65% of all women in Uganda—have at least one problem accessing health care.

A critical development studies framework is needed to unpack the effects of development strategies on the lives of ordinary citizens. This chapter shows that the trust of ordinary citizens has been betrayed repeatedly. Development plans are toothless if they do not ask critical questions. Will development plans result in actions needed to ensure education for all—for both boys and girls and through baccalaureate levels—and literacy for all, both women and men? Will there be access to improved and sustainable water and sanitation sources? What about electricity? Will there be enough food for everyone to eat? Will gainful employment be available to adults who are able to work for pay? Will this work match the skills of the workforce? How reliable will each country's safety net be? A feminist intervention into the critical development studies framework is needed to ensure that gender equity is taken into account in development strategies and to ensure that a rubric of development effectiveness is intentionality to avoid reproducing inequality. Further, this framework insists that multinational corporation actors' and local elites' roles in development are examined critically. To the extent that elites are skimming off the top, and that foreign interests are raping the land and natural resources, analysts must not look the other way. Vigilant appreciative and critical inquiry to consider roles of all actors, as well as adaptive action to adjust development strategies to stamp out exploitation by multinational interests and corruption on the part of elites, is crucial to the success of development plans. In the next chapter, we examine structural and economic impediments to the creation and maintenance of adequate infrastructure for the provision of clean water and safe sanitation technologies in East Africa. And we discuss effects on access to water and sanitation in East Africa.

NOTES

1. This question emanates from a brilliant student in my qualitative methods class in 2016.
2. www.unrefugees.org/where-we-work/south-sudan.
3. From *UNHCR in 2016* (UNHCR 2016a; www.unhcr.org/564da0e00.pdf).
4. From *Global Focus: Uganda* (UNHCR 2017; reporting.unhcr.org/node/5129).
5. From UNHCR 2016b (*Southern Sudan Regional Response Plan*; www.unhcr.org/en-us/partners/donors/589497987/2017-south-sudan-regional-refugee-response-plan-january-december-2017-23.html).
6. Though the UDHS divides this variable into two categories—"physical or sexual" assault—I group both into physical assault, because sexual assault, is, of course, physical. It may be noted that if physical, sexual, and/or emotional assault are grouped, 82% of men with 5 to 6 controlling behaviors and 34% of men exhibiting no (other) marital control behaviors have assaulted their wives (Uganda Bureau of Statistics and Institute for Resource Development/Macro Systems 2011, 262).

Chapter Two

Structural and Economic Analysis of Declines in Water and Sanitation in East Africa

Shorma Bianca Bailey and Assata Zerai

With the widespread settler and administrative colonial presence, European colonialism of the African continent drastically and irreparably changed the sociopolitical and economic structures of the people living in what would become African countries. In this chapter, we begin a discussion of historical and contemporary factors that have led to the maldistribution of safe water and sanitation infrastructure in East Africa. These influences include the uneven development instigated as part of the region's colonial heritage, the influences of multinational corporations, economic structural adjustment programs, the tourism industry, failing development infrastructure, and the incursion of non-governmental organizations. The tables in this chapter provide recent estimates for water and sanitation coverage for Kenya, Tanzania, and Uganda from the World Health Organization (WHO/UNICEF Joint Monitoring Programme for Water Supply and Sanitation 2014, 2015). DHS and other secondary data provide evidence that allows us to paint a vivid picture of decreasing water availability predicated upon the utter breakdown in development resources and infrastructure, the result of both external and internal factors.

The state of water quantity and access to clean water and sanitation in East Africa is linked to economic and physical water scarcity (Molden 2007). Physical water scarcity can be described as limited water supply available with little opportunity for construction of dams or wells (Molden 2007). Governments in the Global South at times lack the economic capacity to provide sustainable infrastructure to address the need for clean water and safe sanitation to all residents (Molden 2007). Infrastructural investments that include building dams, wells, and piping systems to access safe water and sanitation promote the quality of life of residents. Before delving more deeply into the current economic water scarcity of East African countries, we will review historical antecedents to current systems.

THE EARLIEST RECORDS OF METHODS TO CLEAN WATER (1400 B.C. TO 16TH CENTURY)

The Quest for Pure Water chronicles was written by Moses N. Baker, a member of the American Water Works Association. This book described the quest for proven methods and technologies used by the ancient Egyptians and others to maintain sanitary environmental conditions and to purification of water. In the book, Moses N. Baker states, "The earliest recorded knowledge of water treatment, was found in Egyptian inscriptions and Sanskrit medical lore" (Baker 1948, pp. 1–2). It is important to realize that sanitation strategies and technology for water purification existed thousands of years ago, from the beginning of the first civilization up to the 16th century. The Oustruta Sanghita, a collection of medical lore in Sanskrit dating back to 2000 B.C., states a brief method for water purification (Baker 1948). Several water purification techniques are described on page 1 of *The Quest for Pure Water*: "It is good to keep water in a copper vessel, to expose it to sunlight, and filter through charcoal." In approximately 1450 B.C., written records were documented concerning the hieroglyphics on Amenhotep II's tomb at Thebes. The wall of the Pharaoh Amenhotep II's tomb displayed the likeness of two Egyptians siphoning off boiled water or wine, clarified by a sedimentation system pictured in Wilkinson's *Manners and Customs of the Ancient Egyptians* (Wilkinson 1841).

Sanitation in Egypt

In addition to their domestic and agricultural use of water for drinking, washing, cooking, and irrigation, Egyptians have long considered water a sacred and divine substance. The Nile River, sourced in Lake Tana and Lake Victoria in Eastern Africa, runs through present-day Uganda, South Sudan, Sudan, and Ethiopia and eventually all the way through Egypt,[1] splitting the nation into two lands, making the Nile the main source of water for many of the civilizations living in parts of eastern Africa (Wilkinson 1841). The Upper and Lower regions of Egypt benefited from the river's predicted flooding, which infused an abundance of nutrients to the soil, enabling a continuing surplus of crops. The Nile River water was also used to irrigate farmland to support crop growth (Angelakis and Rose 2014).

Historians including Herodotus and Diodorus documented numerous agricultural scenes in the tombs of Thebes and Lower Egypt, displaying representations of agricultural processes including ploughing, hoeing, sowing, reaping, threshing, winnowing, and housing grain (Wilkinson 1841). Although the Nile River provided agricultural advantages to the ancient Egyptians, its cyclical flooding disrupted the soil, leading to erosion and redeposition of sediments. In other words, soil disruptions due to flooding left farmers with damaged or improved soil.

> It is reasonable to suppose that as the inundation subsided, much litigation sometimes occurred between neighbors. The fall of a portion of the bank, carried away by the stream during the rise of the Nile, frequently made great alterations in the extent of land near the river side; we therefore readily perceive the necessity of determining the quantity which belonged to each individual, whether to settle disputes with a neighbor, or to ascertain the tax due to government. (Campbell 1871, p. 1)

Around 3000 B.C., the Pharaoh Menes in his reign constructed a system of canals and channels using prior scientific knowledge. Pharaoh Menes also built sedimentation basins to hold flood water, dug canals, and irrigation water (Angelakis and Rose 2014). During the Ramesside period, following the Bronze Age, Egypt would fall into the hands of its first Greek ruler, called Ptolemy Soter the I. Ptolemy Soter ruled Egypt until 30 B.C., when Egypt was taken by the Roman Empire. Christianity became to make its way into Egypt's polytheistic religion during the reign of Ptolemy Soter I, also known as Serapis. *Encyclopedia Britannica Online* describes a structural device used in Egypt called a *noria*, a water wheel (Christensen 2015). This ancient water transportation device, used to raise water in primitive irrigation systems, was noted by Roman architect Vitruvius in about the 1st century B.C. Water was also used to make skins, paint, and linens and to produce flax for cloth. Perfumes and natural soaps were also processed by women to maintain hygiene and sanitation. The many achievements of the Egyptian civilization include quarrying; surveying; construction techniques that facilitated the building of pyramids and temples; a practical and effective system of medicine and mathematics; irrigation systems and agricultural production techniques; and the earliest known peace treaty. Under the span of Arab, Mameluke, and Ottoman conquests in Egypt, the ancient civilization still maintained national consciousness and remained a separate entity that seemingly became the center for civilization in North and East Africa (Angelakis and Rose 2014).

With respect to early Egyptian water treatment and sanitation, the most documented woman in ancient civilization was the great mathematician-astronomer Hypatia. In the area of water technology Hypatia, the mathematician, invented a device to measure the level of water and designed a distillation apparatus for the boiling of water and another instrument called an aerometer to determine the specific gravity of liquids (Mozans 1913). (Distillation is the process of using heat to separate substances of differences boiling points to obtain a desired purity.) Alongside her many inventions, Hypatia also created an astrolabe and a planisphere. Under the rule of Julius Caesar around 48 B.C., the Library of Alexandria, where Hypatia studied, was burned to the ground. The destruction of the library was a symbol of destruction of religion and science. The religious conflict between Christianity, Neoplatonism and the Traditional Egyptian Spirituality system may have contributed to the burning of the Library of Alexandria. Hypatia, a woman of high intellect, was well regarded as one of the most prominent mathematicians and astronomers in Alexandria during her time. Despite her popularity in the arts and sciences and mathematics, Hypatia's Neoplatonist ideology was seen as "pagan." For a time Hypatia could express her religious freedom and even obtained a substantial following during her lectures. Proceeding the burning of the Library of Alexandria the Serapeum was built. The Serapeum was a symbol to represent the Greco-Egyptian god Serapis or Ptolemy Soter I. Shortly after the rise of Cyril to the bishopric of Alexandria, Hypatia was drug through the streets of Alexandria and murdered at the hands of a gang of Christian zealots. Hypatia the great mathematician and astronomer was a powerful symbol of African feminism and activism. She used her intellect to help improve the quality of life for all peoples during that time of religious persecution, advancement in math, and science. Hypatia's murder was a result of gender inequality, sexism and intersectionality in a prehistoric colonialist society.

Women such as Hypatia played significant roles in the prehistoric society in perpetuating methods of learning, cleanliness, and sanitation for the household. Gender roles documented in literature directly and indirectly suggests the responsibility of the women traditionally included in transporting water for drinking, cooking, washing, bathing, and agriculture.

WOMEN, WATER, AND SANITATION IN CONTEMPORARY EAST AFRICA

Women and girls are traditionally responsible for domestic water supply and sanitation, in addition to maintaining a hygienic home environment (UNICEF 2003). As managers at the household level, women have a high stake in the improvement of water and sanitation services and in sustaining facilities (UNICEF 2003). Furthermore, improvement of water and sanitation conditions is often dependent on the financial state of the household. Policymakers often view educating girls as a way to put countries on the fast track to economic development. Evidence-based research shows that maternal health education is an important antecedent to judicious use of WASH technologies and better child health outcomes. In a study of DHS data from Malawi, Tanzania, and Zimbabwe, Makoka and Masibo (2015) show that the threshold of the amount of maternal education that reduces the level of undernutrition in children is 10 completed years. And in Kenya, the Ministry of Education, Science and Technology has emphasized the important role that education plays in the implementation of water and sanitation policies, stating that high morbidity rates can be lowered by instituting school health and feeding programs to "reinforce provision of safe water and sanitation with health and hygiene promoting education materials" (Republic of Kenya 2008, p. 30). "The correlation between investment in girls' education and economic growth was proliferated by 1980s World Bank research that illustrated how improved access and enrollment of girls in formal schooling led to increased GDP per capita, decreased infant mortality rates and increased life expectancies" (Desai 2016, pp. 250–251).

While NGOs, industry, and others may aim to harness the power of women and girls through country programs that promote the education and equal rights of women to participate freely in the political, social, and economic development of their communities (UNICEF 2003), the focus of these campaigns draws attention away "from increasing global structural inequalities and transnational circuits of power at the individual and systemic level" (Desai 2016, p. 260). Additionally, by positioning these basic rights and public goods as part of national development agendas and policies, benchmarks of success are also economically determined. That is, if girls can access clean water, education, and sanitation, there are no measures in place to determine this as a successful provision of public services. Rather, because of the history of colonialism and the lasting impacts in global economic systems that demand participation as a proxy for advancement, "with the support of international aid agencies, national states such as Bangladesh, India, Kenya, and Indonesia have targeted poor and rural women in the interests of national development" (Puri 2004, p. 115). These long-term goals to increase access to education do little to address the water and sanitation crisis that is currently underway in Kenya, Tanzania, and Uganda. Moreover, the focus on the increase of education to improve livelihoods and health is always monetized and positioned as part of a broader economic agenda. For instance, in Vision 2030, Kenya's social and economic policy in place since 2012, education, health, sanitation, and economic growth are all in service of "making Kenya a newly industrializing, middle income country, providing high quality life for all its citizens by the year 2030" (Kenya Vision 2030, 2016).

This phenomenon is not new, nor is it unique to Kenya. As Karishma Desai explains, it has come to govern national policies, donor requirements, and multinational incentives. However, linkages must be made not only between the enrollment of girls in formal education and better development outcomes, but also between environmental, economic, and structural factors that are closely tied to water and sanitation. For example, the WHO (June 2016) describes the water and sanitation crisis in East Africa due to floods and climatic drought–related conditions caused by El Niño. According to Ibrahima-Soce Fall (2006), the El Niño weather event impacted millions of Eastern Africans, including those in Ethiopia, Tanzania, and Kenya, contaminating many water sources and spreading disease. Food insecurity and severe acute malnutrition have consequently increased significantly in the affected countries. A focus solely on women's education misses other important factors. Below, we examine water coverage and availability of improved sanitation and point to structural and economic factors contributing to changes in these resources over time.

Water Coverage

Tables 2.1, 2.2, and 2.3 detail estimated water sources for Kenya, Tanzania, and Uganda, respectively, for 1990 to 2015. Due to rapid urbanization, water coverage in Kenya's urban areas has declined since 1990. Urban improved sources were 92% then, but this declined to 82% by 2015. Water piped into urban premises has taken the largest hit in the past two decades, declining from 55% of households in 1990 to 45% in 2015. All other improved urban sources were stable in the same period, and access to surface

Table 2.1. Estimated Water Sources in Kenya, 1990–2015

Year	Total Improved (%)	Piped onto Premises (%)	Other Improved (%)	Other Unimproved (%)	Surface Water (%)
			Urban water		
1990	92	55	37	5	3
1995	90	53	37	6	4
2000	87	51	36	9	4
2005	85	49	36	10	5
2010	83	47	36	12	5
2015	82	45	37	13	5
			Rural water		
1990	33	10	23	19	48
1995	38	11	27	18	44
2000	43	11	32	17	40
2005	48	12	36	17	35
2010	53	13	40	16	31
2015	57	14	43	15	28
			Total water		
1990	43	17	26	16	41
1995	47	18	29	16	37
2000	52	19	33	15	33
2005	56	20	36	15	29
2010	60	21	39	15	25
2015	63	22	41	15	22

Source: WHO/UNICEF Joint Monitoring Programme for Water Supply and Sanitation 2014, 2015.

Table 2.2. Estimated Water Sources in United Republic of Tanzania, 1990–2015

Year	*Total Improved (%)*	*Piped onto Premises (%)*	*Other Improved (%)*	*Other Unimproved (%)*	*Surface Water (%)*
			Urban water		
1990	92	31	61	5	3
1995	89	30	59	8	3
2000	86	29	57	11	3
2005	83	29	54	14	3
2010	80	28	52	17	3
2015	77	28	49	20	3
			Rural water		
1990	45	0	45	30	25
1995	45	1	44	31	24
2000	45	2	43	32	23
2005	45	3	42	33	22
2010	45	4	41	34	21
2015	46	6	40	34	20
			Total water		
1990	54	6	48	25	21
1995	54	7	47	26	20
2000	54	8	46	27	19
2005	55	10	45	28	17
2010	55	11	44	29	16
2015	56	13	43	30	14

Source: WHO/UNICEF Joint Monitoring Programme for Water Supply and Sanitation 2014, 2015.

water increased by 2%. Improved coverage has likewise increased steadily since 1990 in rural areas, though the 57% level in 2015 is still less than urban area coverage of 82%. Overall the country's total improved water coverage is 63%. And Kenya's total rate of water piped into premises is 22%, according to WHO/UNICEF Joint Monitoring Programme (WHO/UNICEF Joint Monitoring Programme for Water Supply and Sanitation 2015).

Urban water coverage in Tanzania has also declined, from 92% in 1990 to 77% in 2015 (the latest estimate available from WHO/UNICEF Joint Monitoring Programme for Water Supply and Sanitation 2015). The decline of 15 points was worse than the 10-point decline in Kenya for the same dates. Water piped into residence has declined from 31% in 1990 to 28% in urban areas of Tanzania, and other improved water sources in urban areas have also declined, from 61% in 1990 to 49% in 2015. Unimproved water sources in Tanzania have increased by a factor of 4, from 5% in 1990 to 20% in 2011.

Table 2.3. Estimated Water Sources in Uganda, 1990–2015

Year	*Total Improved (%)*	*Piped onto Premises (%)*	*Other Improved (%)*	*Other Unimproved (%)*	*Surface Water (%)*
			Urban water		
1990	78	7	71	18	4
1995	82	11	71	15	3
2000	85	14	71	12	3
2005	89	17	72	9	2
2010	93	21	72	6	1
2015	96	23	73	3	1
			Rural water		
1990	36	0	36	38	26
1995	44	0	44	33	23
2000	52	1	51	29	19
2005	61	1	60	23	16
2010	69	1	68	19	12
2015	71	1	75	14	10
			Total water		
1990	40	1	39	36	24
1995	48	2	46	32	20
2000	56	2	54	27	17
2005	64	3	61	22	14
2010	73	4	69	16	11
2015	79	5	74	13	8

Source: WHO/UNICEF Joint Monitoring Programme for Water Supply and Sanitation 2014, 2015.

Surface water coverage remains at 3% in urban areas. Rural areas in Tanzania have experienced a very slight increase in total improved water coverage, from 45% in 1990 to 46% in 2015. Other improved sources have increased as well, from 30% in 1990 to 34% in 2015. Finally, in rural areas of Tanzania, water piped into premises has increased from 0% in 1990 to 6% in 2011. Total water coverage in Tanzania has thus increased in regards to total improved water sources and decreased regarding other improved water sources. Water piped into premises in Tanzania has more than doubled, from 6% in 1990 to 13% 2011. Unimproved water sources in Tanzania have also increased from 25% in 1990 to 30% by 2011, and surface water has decreased from 21% in 1990 to 14% in 2011 (WHO/UNICEF Joint Monitoring Programme for Water Supply and Sanitation 2015).

According to the United Republic of Tanzania's Ministry of Water, it established a Big Results Now initiative in May 2013. This initiative describes the instillation of 16,784 water points from July 2013 to June 2014, "benefitting a total of 4.2 million additional people with access to clean safe water supply" (Levira 2016).

Of the three countries, Uganda has most successfully increased its water resources in both urban and rural areas. The total improved sources have increased in urban areas from 78% in 1990 to 96% in 2015, and in rural areas from 36% in 1990 to 76% in 2015. Overall the period of growth from 1990 to 2015 has resulted in 79% of households in rural and urban areas having access to improved water sources. Unimproved water sources have decreased in rural and urban areas. The country's total of unimproved water sources has been reduced from 36% in 1990 to 13% in 2015, despite the decrease in surface water in Uganda from 24% in 1990 to 8% in 2012 (see Table 2.3).

Sanitation

Tables 2.4, 2.5, and 2.6 detail estimated sanitation coverage for Kenya, Tanzania, and Uganda, respectively, for 1990 to 2015. According to the WHO/

Table 2.4. Estimated Sanitation Coverage in Kenya, 1990–2015

Year	*Improved (%)*	*Shared (%)*	*Other Unimproved (%)*	*Open Defecation (%)*
		Urban sanitation		
1990	27	41	29	3
1995	28	42	27	3
2000	29	43	25	3
2005	30	45	22	3
2010	30	46	21	3
2015	31	48	18	3
		Rural sanitation		
1990	24	16	38	22
1995	25	16	38	21
2000	26	17	38	19
2005	28	18	36	18
2010	29	19	36	16
2015	30	19	36	15
		Total sanitation		
1990	25	20	36	19
1995	26	21	36	17
2000	27	22	35	16
2005	28	24	33	15
2010	29	25	33	13
2015	30	27	31	12

Source: WHO/UNICEF Joint Monitoring Programme for Water Supply and Sanitation 2014, 2015.

Table 2.5. Estimated Sanitation Coverage in United Republic of Tanzania, 1990–2015

Year	*Improved (%)*	*Shared (%)*	*Other Unimproved (%)*	*Open Defecation (%)*
		Urban sanitation		
1990	6	6	86	2
1995	11	11	76	2
2000	16	16	66	2
2005	21	21	56	2
2010	26	26	46	2
2015	31	31	36	2
		Rural sanitation		
1990	7	3	80	10
1995	7	3	78	12
2000	7	3	77	13
2005	8	4	74	14
2010	8	4	73	15
2015	8	4	71	17
		Total sanitation		
1990	7	4	80	9
1995	8	5	77	10
2000	9	6	75	10
2005	11	8	70	11
2010	13	10	65	12
2015	16	12	60	12

Source: WHO/UNICEF Joint Monitoring Programme for Water Supply and Sanitation 2014, 2015.

UNICEF Joint Monitoring Programme for Water Supply and Sanitation (2015), improved urban sanitation sources have increased in both Kenya and Tanzania. In Kenya, improved sanitation increased from 26% in 1990 to 31% in 2012. In Tanzania, urban sanitation increased from 9% in 1990 to 24% in 2011. Whereas sanitation increased slightly in urban areas of Kenya, it has almost tripled in urban areas of Tanzania. Open defecation rates in urban areas of Kenya and Tanzania have remained constant at 3% and 2%, respectively. In Uganda, improved sanitation has increased by only 1% in urban areas, though its rate is still higher in urban households than in Kenya and Tanzania. According to WHO/UNICEF (WHO/UNICEF Joint Monitoring Programme for Water Supply and Sanitation 2015), 33% of Uganda's urban households had improved sanitation in 2012. And open defecation remained constant from 1990 to 2012 (2%) in urban Uganda.

In rural areas of Kenya, Tanzania, and Uganda, improved sanitation for households has increased, though by varying degrees. Kenya's increase is

Table 2.6. Estimated Sanitation Coverage in Uganda, 1990–2015

Year	*Improved (%)*	*Shared (%)*	*Other Unimproved (%)*	*Open Defecation (%)*
		Urban sanitation		
1990	28	43	27	2
1995	28	43	27	2
2000	28	43	27	2
2005	28	43	27	2
2010	28	44	26	2
2015	29	44	25	2
		Rural sanitation		
1990	11	6	61	22
1995	13	6	62	19
2000	14	7	63	16
2005	15	8	64	13
2010	16	8	66	10
2015	17	9	66	8
		Total sanitation		
1990	13	10	57	20
1995	14	11	58	17
2000	16	11	58	15
2005	17	12	59	12
2010	18	13	60	9
2015	19	14	60	7

Source: WHO/UNICEF Joint Monitoring Programme for Water Supply and Sanitation 2014, 2015.

5% (24% in 1990; 29% in 2012), Tanzania's increase is 1% (6% in 1990; 7% in 2011), and Uganda's 9% increase is the most impressive of the three countries (25% in 1990; 34% in 2012). Open defecation has increased only in Tanzania's rural areas, from 10% to 16% in 2011; in Kenya it has decreased from 22% to 17% and in Uganda from 22% to 9%. By the latest available estimates (WHO/UNICEF Joint Monitoring Programme for Water Supply and Sanitation 2015) of overall improved sanitation for households, the rates are 30% in Kenya, 12% in Tanzania, and 34% in Uganda.

So what accounts for Uganda's relative success in increasing improved urban and rural water, for its most increased improved rural sanitation, and for its slow increases in improved urban sanitation? And what accounts for Kenya's urban improved water decreases, impressive rural improved water increases, and slow increases in improved sanitation? Finally, what accounts for Tanzania's improved water decreases, impressive urban sanitation increases, and slow rural sanitation increases? How do recent geopolitical and economic factors affect the availability of clean water and improved sanitation? What inequalities are created by current water and sanitation technologies? And how do African feminist perspectives shed light on the problem? Chapters in this book address these issues. But in the following, we explore Uganda's success.

Drill Down: Uganda

Uganda is on target to meet the sustainable development goal of ensuring environmental sustainability; of particular note is its work toward decreasing "the proportion of people without sustainable access to safe drinking water and basic sanitation" (Ministry of Finance, Planning and Economic Development 2013, p. iii). Uganda's Ministry of Finance (Ministry of Finance, Planning and Economic Development 2013) has focused investments on increasing access to safe water and sanitation in rural areas. The indicator of success is that by 2015, 77% of households had access to an improved water source. As mentioned above, the 2012 estimated coverage of total improved water coverage is 95% in urban areas and 71% in rural areas (PMA 2015). And the proportion of households using an improved sanitation facility is 13% (PMA 2015). Achieving improved water access has been more challenging; rates are currently 33% in urban areas and 34% in rural areas for utilizing improved sanitation facilities. Equitable distribution of sanitation among rural and urban areas has resulted in rural areas' 9-point increase from 1990 to 2012. But Uganda still has a long way to go.

The Ministry of Finance admits that, though access to clean water has improved along with some other millennium development goals (MDGs),[2] collecting water, economic activities, and other aspects of life still reproduce gender inequality. Greater gender equality in the education system has been slow to translate into the economic and social spheres.

> Gender inequalities are evident in patterns of time use. On average women work seven hours a week less than men in economic activities (working for pay or profit, or contributing to a family business or farm), but significantly more in homecare activities (the collection of firewood and fetching of water, construction of own dwellings and farm building, milling and other food processing for own consumption). Women are more likely than men to work low-value-added primary activities, accounting for 55% of the workforce in the agriculture, forest and fishing sector in 2009/10. Of the women working outside of the agricultural sector, 62% are employed in the informal sector compared to 55% of men. (Ministry of Finance, Planning and Economic Development 2013, p. 21)

While examining rural and urban differences in access to water and sanitation is helpful, it is important to consider differences between provinces, and most especially differences even within the confines of one city. Katanga, an informal settlement area within Kampala, can be found "sandwiched between Makerere University and Mulago Hospital—both institutions are the city's rare epitome of progressive development. . . . Located about 2 kilometers from Kampala's city center," Katanga is like another world (Matubaazi 2006). An informant notes, "Here we don't have bathrooms. So people just shower from their verandas because there is no space to build bathrooms" (Matubaazi 2006). In 2006, the population of the Katanga settlement area was reportedly 16,000. It is characteristics of other informal settlement areas such as Kamwokya, Makerere Kivulu, Banda, Wabigalo, Namuwongo, Kalerwe, Nsambya and Bwaise, and other districts including Jinja, Mbale and Gulu and Namuwongo, where open sewage includes "dead animals like dogs, cats, and chicken to human waste" (Matubaazi 2006). The World Bank estimates that over 60% of the urban population of Uganda lives in such unplanned settlement areas (Lall 2015). Residents of areas pool resources, and many belong to the National Slum Dwellers Federation of Uganda (NSDFU): "Founded in 2002, the NSDFU today comprises almost 500 savings groups and approximately 38,000 members. Savings are used to bring people together, build their capacity to act collectively, and build organizational capacity and trust" (World Bank 2013, 115).

A reported 44,600 people live in Uganda's unplanned settlements (Harris, n.d.). "The drainage channel reduces in size at some points because of obvious encroachment by human activities. At one point, it disappears into a household emerging out at a doorstep of another household. Here, residents improvise by putting barriers across the channel to allow them to move in and out of their residences" (Matubaazi 2006).

Relationality is evident, as part of the contamination of water resources in the Namuwongo slums comes from "a combination of industrial waste and the run-off from the high lying areas of Kampala" (Beauvoisin 2013). "The majority of the slum's population comes from the war-torn zones of Northern Uganda, Congo and Rwanda. Others have migrated from Kenya using the railway line" (Beauvoisin 2013). Several improvements have been made in unplanned settlement areas over the past few years—some resulting from resident organizing and savings clubs, others coming from NGOs such as Hope for Children—and the Uganda government has invested in building infrastructure for these areas.

Residents explain their experiences. And news reports (Ogwang 2013) provide context.

> Life in the slums is not any cheap, though. While water coverage in Kampala, for example, is estimated at 65%, it costs three times more to buy water in a city slum than it does in the planned areas such as Kololo and Nakasero, a Kampala Integrated Environmental Planning Management Project (KIEMP),

> 2010, report [cited in Ogwang 2013] says that . . . "A UN-habitat observatory report, 2007, ranked Uganda among developing countries with fast annual slum growth rate, averaging 5.32%, implying there are about 3.5 million Ugandans living in slums today, estimated to reach eight million by 2020, up from three million in 2009."

Such reports also provide hope. "In her quest to curtail the slum problem, Uganda developed the National Slum Upgrading Strategy and Action Plan . . . to provide a framework, direction and plan to all stakeholders on how to improve slums. This would fast-track Uganda's target of uplifting the lives of at least one million people by 2020" (Ogwang 2013). Other examples of activism to promote the welfare of residents in unplanned settlements include The Transforming Settlements of Urban Poor in Uganda (TSUPU) program, which has also been developed to mobilize slum dwellers in Kampala, Jinja, Mbale, Arua, Mbarara, and Kabaale into forming savings groups through slum dwellers' federations.

> TSUPU, funded partly from a World Bank-based Cities Alliance grant, seeks to guide balanced urbanization by creating regional cities, says Mabala, adding that through the Community Upgrading Fund, the Government plans to give small grants of between sh10–sh30m to help improve infrastructure services. The three-year (2011–13) sh637 m [*Ed:* 637 million Tanzanian shillings] scheme will ensure Arua, Jinja, Mbale, Mbarara and Kabaale get sh200 m to improve their infrastructures, especially drainages, annually. (Ogwang 2013)

ADDRESSING GENDER INEQUALITY IN EAST AFRICA

Educational and societal norms often limit the ability for women and girls to become paid skilled laborers (Jansz and Wilbur 2013). As a result, women and girls, by society, are not seen as an economic powerhouse. Gender inequality continues to be perpetuated when women are not credited for their contributions to society. Empowering women and girls through education, opportunity for economic impact, and health education can potentially contribute to an improved quality of life for them and their families (United Nations 2010).

While progress has been made toward achieving the UN Millennium Development Goals (MDGs), the progress has not yielded equitable results—sizable gender gaps still exist (World Bank 2011). Hypothetically, considering the potential for gender parity to be achieved, the question must be asked, Would GDP then be a function of the gender parity parameters? In September 2015, McKinsey Global Institute (MGI) published a study on gender parity and its residual effects on global gross domestic product. Data was obtained from 95 countries, including East African countries Kenya and Tanzania categorized under sub-Saharan Africa. Two scenarios were assumed. The first was a "full potential" or "equal opportunity" scenario where women had participation in the economy that equal to men. The second case was a "business as usual" approach, which is the current state. In the current state of economics, women make up only one-third of the workforce, the other two-thirds are populated by males. The scenario involving women at an equal level of participation with men resulted in a $28 trillion annual global GDP in 2025 and a 26% financial increase compared with the current state of business. This substantial growth in GDP is almost as large as the economies of China and the United States combined. However, educating girls alone will not achieve such results. It is important to address gender inequity at all levels.

Another case study conducted was called "best-in-region." In this case countries matched their rate of improvement compared to the best-performing country in their region. In following this scenario, the potential addition to the annual GDP in 2025 is an estimated $12 trillion, which is almost equivalent to the combined GDPs of Japan, Germany, and the United Kingdom. Assigning a monetary value to gender equality as it relates to employment further validates and sheds light on the dollar value of women's working. Proving that the global economics is a function of the female work force is very difficult, yet MGI's research demonstrated this effort through reporting the gender parity score. Gender parity, an index released by UNESCO, is a socioeconomic index that measures the quotient of the number of females over the number of men enrolled at a given stage of education. Troubled areas where females are most deprived of gender equity are in areas of the Middle East and North Africa as measured by a Gender Parity Score (GPS), which measures the distance each country has traveled toward gender parity, which is set at 1.00. In the Middle East and North Africa the GPS is 0.48; in India 0.48; in South Asia (excluding India) 0.44; and in sub-Saharan Africa 0.57, compared with developed regions such as North America (0.74) and Western Europe (0.71) (McKinsey Global Institute 2015). This analysis from 95 countries determined that the regional economic output generated by women in North America, China, Eastern Europe, and Central Asia is about 40%, whereas Middle East and North Africa account for 18% of female economic output.

The study presented by MGI emphasizes the dependency of a nation's economy on the progression of poverty and education. Women's and girls' limited access to education may affect the overall economic status quo. This trend may also reveal other inferences about countries with low gender parity scores. One inference is that low gender parity is potentially indicative of poverty, whereas a higher, more proportioned gender parity score closer to 1 would indicate a wealthier economic country. In other words, poverty is a factor that is influenced by education and vice versa. It is also imperative to briefly discuss the progress of the educational systems in East Africa. Higher education in Tanzania, Kenya, and Uganda is necessary for economic growth as well as for improved quality of life. Females are less likely than males to attend a college or university in these parts of the world. Not only do gender inequality and poverty factors influence the quality of higher education, but the internationalization of education leaves Africa at a disadvantage in the global higher education network. However, most gender parity parameters focus on primary and less often secondary education. The need for women to obtain higher education and address tremendous gaps by gender is under discussed.

WOMEN, WATER, AND SANITATION TO IMPROVE ECONOMIC POWER

Women played significant roles in the prehistoric society, especially in the transport of water, purification of water, and maintenance of safe sanitation. Women such as Hypatia in ancient Alexandria, Egypt, have also contributed knowledge to aid in the purification and management of water. Women are the backbone of the household in places like Tanzania, Kenya, and Uganda and sometimes are not afforded the same opportunities for education as boys because of culture and tradition.

Traditionally women have overseen the inner workings of the household; they established and maintained household methods of cleanliness and sanitation. However, documentation of women and their role in water in prehistoric times is sparse, aside from references to women being the main transporters of water to the household for drinking, cooking, washing, bathing, and agriculture. In the 35 countries, today, women are more than twice as likely than men to collect drinking water (World Health Organization 2006). Resulting from lack of access to piped water, a daily task for some females in rural areas of Tanzania, Kenya, and Uganda is spending more than 30 minutes to collect water. "About 157 million people in the Eastern and Southern Africa region (ESAR) are not connected to a clean and safe water distribution system, and thus need to use external water sources" (UNICEF 2016, p. 1).

Methodologies to improve access to clean water and safe sanitation are consistently undermined by Western gender ideologies of women's roles and economic potential. And it is important to place the shortcomings of the development infrastructure in Kenya, Tanzania, and Uganda in global context; technological advances in those countries are slow to be developed due to economic limitations, limited locally available resources, and often-siloed local knowledge regimes. Through providing accessible educational and occupational opportunities for women and girls, policymakers and activists in East Africa may enhance possibilities for integration of local knowledge with global technologies and empower women and girls to fight for universal access to improved water and sanitation. While globalization is often considered a recent phenomenon, it is nothing new to previously colonized parts of the world, such as the African continent. The remnant of colonialism is apparent. Colonialism strips a people of its culture, freedom, individuality, and, most importantly, self-reliance and empowerment. East African countries were colonialized, resulting in a forced dependency of their peoples to look to the colonial rulers to establish the standard resources and technologies by which to build infrastructure and achieve economic advance. While colonialism specifically hindered women and impeded girls' access to education, it also supported knowledge regimes that are centered on European versions of history and idealized European culture.

In the next chapter, Brenda N. Sanya examines surprising results that come from traditional postcolonial educational practices in Kenya and make recommendations for the types of liberating education that will yield paradigm shifts in our thinking about designing and implementing development infrastructure.

NOTES

1. The word *Egypt* means "two lands." Around 5000 B.C., Egypt was one of the most powerful civilizations that arose along the Nile River Valley (Wilkinson 1841).

2. As noted in the introduction, *Transforming Our World: The 2030 Agenda for Sustainable Development* (https://sustainabledevelopment.un.org/post2015/transformingourworld; United Nations 2015) includes sustainable development goals (SDGs) and multiple indicators of progress. SDGs are an update to the original millennium development goals (MDGs), which ended in 2015. Here we refer to MDGs because the cited report predates 2015.

Chapter Three

Public Goods, Citizenship Rights

How Lingering Structural Inequalities Define Social Services and Government Policies

Brenda N. Sanya

What might education and its role in everyday life tell us about water, sanitation, and healthcare for the women in rural Kenya? The Constitution of Kenya (2010) not only codified rights but also established an equalization fund to be used in part to provide and expand "basic services including water, roads, health facilities and electricity to marginalised areas to the extent necessary to bring the quality of those services in those areas to the level generally enjoyed by the rest of the nation" (The Constitution of Kenya 2010, Article 204). To understand not only how public goods and citizenship rights are distributed in a rural community in Kenya but also the impacts of economic development in shaping national policies, this chapter highlights a disjuncture between what is stipulated in national laws and policies and the actual implementation of those same policies in a rural community that has historically experienced challenges with poor health, education, and sanitation infrastructure and services. In particular, evidence from a study in rural Kenya suggests that high levels of education generate more docile subject-citizens than do lower levels of education, a finding contrary to the claim that education is necessarily emancipatory.

In addition to the constitution, the other significant sociopolitical and economic policy that drives government spending is Kenya's Vision 2030. Paying close attention to the interconnected policies that define social and economic rights, it is evident that Vision 2030's policies around education, health, and social services reinforce western systems and innovations as part of a wider development policy. Introduced in 2008, Vision 2030's developmental blueprint stated a goal to "transform Kenya into a newly industrializing, middle-income country providing a high quality of life to all its citizens by 2030 in a clean and secure environment." This ambitious policy plan targets "economic, social, and political pillars" (Government of the Republic of Kenya 2007, p. 1) that center economic growth and industrialization as the basis for the provision of public goods. Formulated as a plan to be implemented in five-year terms, Vision 2030 centers development as the reason for providing public services to citizens.

In fact, citizenship often takes center stage, as the location where laws and social contacts intersect and ostensibly secure the rights of individuals in relation to the state. Education is often complicit in fortifying the neoliberal logics of the state, being embedded in what critical theorist Keguro Macharia (2017) has termed a "development imaginary." Development as invoked and applied in this sense is bolstered by the social pillars of Vision 2030, which position education and schooling as sites that aim to introduce, create, and secure "compliance and complicity" on behalf of development. As such, it embodies "law-invoking term, a disciplinary term" (see Macharia 2017). For instance, education policy in Vision 2030 aims to provide "globally competitive quality education and training and research for development" (Government of the Republic of Kenya 2007). This ostensibly noble goal also implicitly bulwarks and sustains a discourse of economic development without fostering any questioning around systems of government or the adequate provision of citizenship rights.

In this way, the terms for which education are invoked and introduced into schools and curricula are driven not by critical thinking or to contextualize history as a way to understand contemporary realities, but instead largely focus simply on technocratic, school-based literacy. While potentially increasing the transition rate from primary to secondary schools, and implying that the quality and relevance of education is a stipulated goal, there is no clear evidence of education being anything than what it was under colonial rule: a site of governance and discipline. Despite the potential of education to be liberatory, schooling, when imbricated in state ideologies and global neoliberalism, becomes cruelly optimistic (Berlant 2011). That is, as an optimistic institution, schooling not only constructs subjects and positions them in relationship to the state, but generates a discourse of hope and effort, which, in the vast majority of cases, are not realizable due to existing social inequalities that are further reinforced by neoliberal education. When evoked, this kind of optimism opens us to the promise of schooling as affording better futures. It is the conceptual glue that haphazardly transforms a chaotic world into a space made livable through its embedded hope, even as only a very few find that promise made good on. Consequently, this chapter focuses on some of the multiplicity of roles that education takes up with regard to citizenship, troubling the notions around what constitutes education/educative practices within and beyond the school.

FROM COLONIALISM TO INDEPENDENCE: PUBLIC GOOD, SOCIAL SERVICES, AND GOVERNMENT POLICIES

Scholars of education have documented the perils of an assumption that education is always directly linked to schooling and that education is emancipatory. Rejecting the idea that education—i.e., the process of receiving instruction at an institution—is inherently emancipatory, I show how existing indigenous and customary systems of learning in Kenya can provide solutions that are relevant to improving the lives of people, and women in particular. Even though contemporary international aid and development rhetoric about Africa regard formal education from kindergarten through university schooling as a tool that fosters empowerment, liberation, and agency, I argue that colonial and postcolonial education instead disadvantage women because they entrench and normalize gendered ideologies and the gendered social structure. Thus, the higher the level of their education and the more deeply embedded in their cultures, the more likely women are to cling to existing structures of inequality normalized by the processes of learning. As an outgrowth of colonial civilizing and westernizing schools, education in Kenya valorizes, prioritizes, sometimes unquestioningly privileges, and typically entrenches western innovation and international developments on health, sanitation, and water distribution as sites of advancement.

Education is protected by numerous global/local jurisdictions as a social good. However, from targeted qualitative interviews and government records on rural women living in the Nyanza province of Kenya, it is evident that otherwise rosy assessments concerning the unqualified good of education fail to speak to the lived experiences of many rural community women. For instance, in one community where I conducted a qualitative study to gain insights into women's experiences as they accessed social services, I found that the education provided at public schools in the area served as a sexist and repressive tool that limited women's ability to critically examine their social conditions and the hierarchies created by contemporary, historical, indigenous, and colonial political and religious authorities.

For instance, historical and contemporary political economies continue to bear a strong imprint on the lives of Kenyan women. British colonial conquest, and decades of occupation, led to loss of sovereignty for a majority of Kenyans as colonial leaders replaced the country's indigenous leaders. Moreover, to understand the contemporary through the lens of a history of colonialism and neocolonial arrangements (Spivak 1999, 2004), one must also consider how British colonial economic policy included land alienation, which transferred land from indigenous populations to European settlers, along with African taxation and African migrant/forced labor development

(Sorrenson 1965, Zeleza 1992). This policy, of course, aimed to benefit the British settler community in its quest to improve agricultural production and peasant commodity production for export. Improving this rate of production meant an increased need for a healthy, skilled labor force, more modes of transport to hasten exports, and general infrastructure, including health, sanitation, education, transport, and communication. Not only were these innovations based strictly on Western ideals, they were also provided in earnest only in those areas where the colonialists benefited directly (especially in cities). More simply, these infrastructures were not built with the benefit of Kenyans in mind.

Thus led by the British colonial machinery, Kenya experienced the introduction of forced taxation and entry into wage labor. This process served to reconfigure indigenous networks of social relations and also transformed the ways that social services were provided within Black Kenyan communities. In examining the provision of social services in the division of rural Kenya, I observed how Kenya's colonial history and the industrial revolution in Europe shaped economic policies at my research site in Kenya. The British, in search of mineral and agricultural resources, focused all economic, social, and political activities in Kenya on capitalist interests. Beyond the need for resources to continue industrializing, the basic underlying principle for legitimizing colonialism was based on the assumption that the indigenous populations lacked modernized civilizations. As such, the British colonial regime devoted minimal infrastructure and social services to "civilize" black Kenyans while attempting to maximize economic gain.

Prior to colonialism, Kenya's societies were complex ethnic nationalities structured around a system of chieftaincy led by clan elders. These ethnic nationalities met most welfare requirements of people through communal reciprocity, with little or no monetary exchange (Waris et al. 2009). Legislation introduced by the British colonial government introduced new economic systems with coercive policies—such as the distinction between the homestead and the community, which came about as part of the collection of taxes—and the promotion of money as a primary social currency. By these means, colonialism altered the ethnic sociopolitical landscape of Kenya and permanently eroded the social-support mechanisms originally in place.

As the British industrialization project developed and required greater funding and resources, a policy of fiscal self-sufficiency forced colonial states to rely on locally generated tax revenue. That is, with the introduction of taxation, the cost of this increased funding for production for the British government was dependence on settler and indigenous labor. In 1901, the Hut Tax Regulation inaugurated the most widespread form of revenue collection. This was a property tax, paid for dwelling, and levied on both the settler and indigenous populations. This legislation and its tax obligations ensured that more young, indigenous men (and in some cases women) entered the monetary economy (Waris et al. 2009).

Prior to colonial "modernization," Kenyan communities had social structures, laws, systems of governance, education, and health care that allowed most households to maintain high standards of sanitation. These systems were interrupted by British colonialism. The British colonialists devalued, undermined, and disrupted the indigenous Kenyans' economic and political structures, organizations, and civilizations. They promoted British social, cultural, and economic supremacy, focusing all welfare activities on meeting the needs and interests of the nonindigenous population only (MacPherson 1982). The welfare of Africans was subordinated to that of the colonialists and was considered in utilitarian terms only, to the extent that it benefited colonialists as well. In healthcare, for example, the colonial government established rudimentary hospitals and clinics for the general population, out of a need by European enterprises for healthy workers and to prevent the spread of communicable diseases to colonialists; such hospitals thus were not distributed evenly across the whole of Kenya but only in those areas most settled by colonialists. A similar policy was applied to education, where White children were guaranteed full primary and secondary schooling, in contrast to Black children, especially rural ones.

The effects of the forced taxation, entry into the wage-labor market, and migration to plantations drastically changed the lifestyles of indigenous Kenyans, including by redefining gender roles and breaking down the subsistence farming economy. Families were often split up by migration, with men leaving women, children, and the elderly. This meant that the population left had to take on new roles and replace the labor of absentee sons, husbands, and fathers. In cases where nuclear families migrated for work, they still had to deal with the change from the traditional African extended family to the Western nuclear family. This led to the reduction of communal food production and, in some cases, widespread malnutrition and poverty-related disease.

Specifically, the introduction of land privatization, monetary relations, and the commodification of food production changed how people of the Luo ethnic group lived. The changes were particularly noticeable in the distribution of farm labor—the shift from subsistence farming and fishing to small-scale farming for trade—with women having a diminished role in agricultural production (Ogot 1967). With migration to plantations and urban areas, women's roles in the household and in farming changed, with men's roles taking on a monetized value.

This European model and vision of farm work was distinctly different from farming systems in Africa, where the provision of food was not always the domain of men. Rather, African women had always played a fundamental role in agriculture. Boserup's (1970) analysis of the African shifting agricultural system, which she termed a "female" system of farming, found that colonialism and the penetration of capitalism into subsistence economies contributed to the loss of African women's status. The colonial land reform processes, based on the European culture and practice where cultivation was men's work, led to women's loss of land rights, exacerbated further by the development of plantations and the introduction of European farming systems that influenced migration patterns.

In 1960, the British government accepted the "one person, one vote" principle, and White settlers began to lose some of their political privilege, leading eventually to a Black majority government in 1963. And while colonialism is often conceived as having ended with the introduction of Black indigenous leadership, the Fanonian call for a decolonization of the mind was quickly brushed aside and Kenya's leadership began to transform while still maintaining the previous geopolitical and biopolitical systems of governance. That is, through the maintenance and expansion of the social amenities, educational systems, and infrastructure introduced by White settlers and the colonial government, formerly colonized areas were ontologically transformed. Tuck and Yang explain, "Settlers become the law, supplanting Indigenous laws and epistemologies" (2012, p. 7). Even after new laws were introduced with independence, colonized areas were already transformed, with a share of colonial wealth re-distributed or transferred to national leaders of the newly formed independent nations (see Razack 2002, Tuck and Yang 2012, Kauanui 2016, Jafri 2017). In the Kenyan context, customary law was maintained, but national constitutional law was enforced. Similarly, education in ethnic languages was introduced, but English remained as the primary language of instruction (see Gachukia and Akivaga 1978; Akivaga and Odaga 1983; and Thiong'o 1986). Innovations in health and sanitation remained West-centric. Most significantly, economic development, and the production of surplus, defined success and development overall and currently remains so as the primary policy for Kenya's future. Vision 2030, with its language focused on human lives as a "social strategy" and interested in "investing in the people of Kenya," exemplifies this emphasis. It is in this light and history that I will address education, health, and sanitation.

The new gender division of labor devalued reproductive labor and appointed men as the principal agricultural producers. Consequently, African women's involvement in food cultivation generated a pattern of predominantly male migration, leaving women and children in the village (see Mbilinyi 1996). After colonial occupation ended, the postcolonial government inherited a capitalist model of land distribution and a plantation economy. The Kenyan government also inherited a social service infrastructure instituted by the British that was rudimentary, or in some cases nonexistent. In addition to the influence of economy, culture, and social services, postcolonial Kenyan was governed under a constitution, drafted by 65 nominated members of the legislative council present at three preindependence conferences at Lancaster House, where the first Kenyan constitution was written, debated, and instituted.

With this legacy, political independence did not, perhaps even could not, solve many of the challenges facing Kenya, including unequal land distribution, the exclusion of women from political and economic activity, and limited access to social services. Through limited land reform and restitution of land that had been possessed and occupied by the White settlers, some members of the black elite, who make up only 5% of the population, occupied a majority of land that had once been owned by the colonial government. Many of the displaced indigenous populations remained squatters on the plantations, with the continued presence of White settlers or the transfer of land to black elites. In brief, Kenyan independence involved a transfer of power from the White colonial government to a population of educated, empowered Black elites. In that process, neocolonialism has continued to inform policy by normalizing, reifying, and reproducing Western values, policies, and agendas as circulated through globalization (see Rizvi and Lingard 2000 on the role of colonialism in the global context).

Along with this transfer and maintenance of colonial systems, vestiges of colonialism are found in social structures as well. For instance, prior to colonialism, African households were able to maintain high standards of sanitation, but this changed when all societal systems were reconfigured based on British colonial government needs and standards—often very abruptly, within a single generation, and in unsustainable ways that contribute to the breakdowns that remain today. Present-day Kenya experiences an uncomfortable sociocultural admixture of precolonial, colonial, and global structures. In particular, the postcolonial state has circumvented racial politics and ethnicized the state through the mobilization of the citizenry around ethnic political parties. In a fundamental sense, postcolonial governance has maintained, normalized, and localized patterns of British imperial, autocratic rule.

THE CONFLUENCE OF COLONIALISM AND PATRIARCHY: EDUCATION FOR CIVILIZATION, ASSIMILATION, AND DEVELOPMENT

All of the women in the study, like a majority of the residents of the rural area under study, are subsistence farmers. Economically, apart from subsistence agriculture, some of the residents also engage in small-scale businesses, with a small proportion engaged in casual labor from time to time in agriculture and construction work. The main road in the area is an all-weather road. Additionally, according to a website of Kenya's Ministry of Health (Government of the Republic of Kenya 2010), the local health center—run, funded, and staffed by the government—provides "antenatal, curative outpatient services, family planning, growth monitoring and promotion for infants, HIV counseling and testing, home based care, immunization, and prevention of mother to child transmission of HIV services."

My field research began as a study of how politically generated and culturally engrained conceptions of gender impact whether Luo women in Kenya use health facilities—specifically, health, nutrition, and sanitation services—how often they use the health facilities, and whether they implement recommended preventative health programs. The study therefore was aimed at venturing deeply into the experiences of women in a rural Luo community.

The responses from in-depth interviews with each participant represent the views and experiences of those who participated in the study and raise questions that elaborated on quantitative data gathered from government demographics and statistics. While the results of the interviews were not intended to represent larger populations of rural women all over Kenya, they reflect information that is consistent with domains of other academic inquiry on Kenya, especially with regard to marriage, the role of women, and women's rights.

By an examination of past and existing projects in the area, I developed a research survey designed to collect information in three categories: community perspectives, focusing on understanding tribal power structures and hierarchies in the community; understanding the structural challenges faced by the community in accessing health care; and gender roles and women's rights in both the nation and the community, specifically asking questions about premarital sex, polyandry and polygyny, bride wealth, education of children, land rights, and women's legal rights. I also collected demographics on age, sex, marital status, number of dependents, and education. These demographic markers later proved influential in transforming my research questions. In addition, I had a small sample size: 30 women between the ages of 18 and 68, with 18 of them having less than 5 years of formal education and 12 having more than 5.

The women in this study live in a jurisdiction that was once part of Siaya district and that, for the decade preceding the study, had the highest HIV/AIDS infection rates in Kenya. The district also hosted the first Millennium Village Project (MVP) at Bar Sauri. The guiding principle of the MVP is an integrated approach that works toward a collective improvement of education, health, and sanitation as a way to end the poverty trap. Through this integrated system, problems with education also emerge as challenges to enhanced access to water and improved sanitation.

Specifically, the Bar Sauri MVP uses a comprehensive approach toward eliminating poverty, gender inequality, illness, and disease by improving access to clean water, primary education, basic health care, sanitation, and improved crop production. This also includes distribution of better seeds, fertilizer, and agricultural education. The MVP provided women in this study with farming, nutrition, and health care education.

As Wanjala and Muradian (2013) explain, MVPs were founded on an assumption that targeted public sector investments in a few small-scale venues would increase private savings and that a combination of interventions, "a 'big push' of basic investments in natural assets [. . . ,] health-based interventions [, and . . .] interventions [would] shift to another state in which further development would not depend on external support" (p. 147). Bar Sauri, and the 60,000 people in the surrounding catchment area, was selected for an MVP due to its having vast natural resources needed for sustainable subsistence farming while lacking the revenue for basic services necessary to sustain economic growth; most households practicing subsistence or sub-subsistence farming, for example, injected close to $7 million in the first year alone (Millennium Villages 2010). That increase, as well as the proximity and active participation of the first of the MVP and the local prevalence of HIV/AIDS-related diseases, created a new set of priorities in the region.

Moreover, my familiarity with the region presented unique challenges and opportunities as an outsider-within (Collins 1986). Being fluent in the indigenous language of the region allowed me to gain unique perspectives into community concerns. However, though I had the privilege to gain insights into the community concerns about local government, I also had the responsibility to highlight the "social border spaces occupied by groups of unequal power" (Collins 1998, 5). A central aim of this study was thus to understand how women in the study community conceptualize gender and how they interact with workers of, and resources in, the local health care system. I examined this through in-depth interviews and short surveys designed to assess wait times—including in comparison to government-prescribed policies and practices—poor treatment, and the gender and class climate, as well as the concerns of the women, specifically as regards health.

During the transcription and analysis of my results, I noticed that the women with the lowest levels of formal education were questioning their rights and their marginalization in positions of leadership and were expressing an awareness of the injustice surrounding their negative treatment at health facilities. Even more striking were those who had more than 5 years of schooling reporting injustice with a sense of complacency and acceptance. This last, counterintuitive result emerged also in participants with a tertiary education. This sparked questions around the emancipatory claims of education and the functional role of education in this community, particularly in the face of data otherwise showing the positive effects of education surrounding health and nutrition.

Thus even if, according to the 2014 Kenya Demographic and Health Survey, the "percentage of women and men with no education has dropped by half over the last 10 years, from 13 percent and 6 percent in 2003 to 7 percent and 3 percent, respectively" (Kenya National Bureau of Statistics (KNBS) and ICF Macro 2015, p. xxi), it became even more imperative to interrogate the policy-influencing ideologies at play, especially in light of assumptions that Western civilization, international agenda initiatives, and access to basic education would eliminate women's gendered oppression (Prieto 2010).

While we agree that education for both boys and girls is necessary, in countries without gender parity, appropriate resources must be allocated to ensure that girls and women have equal access to education. We must be cautious, then, that the valorization of education and the push for universal primary education (UPE) as a global development goal not evade or ignore questions of content and the ways that education can function and continues to function as an ideological state apparatus for circulating nationalist agendas that imply or require second-class citizenship for women. For example, the argument that advancing gender parity is a disadvantage to men is consistently used by "men's rights activists" to advance a claim that the education of girls and women is intended to make men submissive. This is simply one face of the prevailing ideological state apparatus that aims at reproducing citizen-subjects able to meet global economic demands by propagating racialized and gendered ideologies that mandate the life trajectories of women while also eliminating existing indigenous, non-Western technologies that have not been proven to be inferior, such as the replacement of traditional pit latrines with flush toilets without sustainable access to water and sewage systems. It is this ideological assumption around the Western, the civilized, and the patriarchal, along with its concomitant erasure of traditional health, sanitation, and water distribution practices, that this study challenges.

BIOGRAPHICAL SKETCHES

From the results of data analysis that showed a disjunction between education and liberation, I selected three women—pseudonymously Auma, Achieng', and Awino—whose responses especially signaled this disjunction. These sketches, distilled from interviews, provide insights about their experiences with learning, schooling, health services, and social amenities. All three live within the catchment area of the local health center and the MVPs clinic; they all visit the same clinic. The experiences documented in the following excerpts recount experiences at this local clinic. Some of the details, especially surrounding education and acts of injustice, are vague or intentionally omitted in order to protect the women's anonymity.

Auma

At the time of our first interview, Auma was 52 years old. She had been widowed at age 30. At the time of her husband's death, they had 4 children. Following his death, Auma had 2 more children, conceived via the traditional custom of wife inheritance. At the time when Auma attended primary school, education was neither free nor compulsory. She attended for 4 years, learning to read, write, and do basic arithmetic; she has since attended one adult education course to improve her arithmetic skills. Auma is part of a nonreligious women's collective focused on improving the status of local women and improving the lives of people living in the community. In her interview, Auma gave extensive answers, highlighting her experiences, disappointments, and hopes. She asserts there is no meaningful difference between boys and girls educationally; she thinks that both her sons and daughters have the same aptitude. Nonetheless, her youngest daughter could not attend school due to tuition costs. Auma repeatedly mentioned that she wishes she could have afforded to send her daughter to school, that she would have educated all of her children, although she also thinks that it is more important to educate girls.

According to Auma, the most powerful person in her village is a government official. This person, usually a man, is called a village elder. Auma has previously been nominated to the position but declined because, she said, "The position needs to be a man because at night when you arrest men, they may attack you." If Auma were a man, she says, would accept this position or similarly a position of leadership in the church. She also spoke of furthering her education, if she were a man. In decision making, Auma is fearless, having been widowed at such a young age and having to care for 6 children. She pointed out that she goes to the hospital or the clinic whenever she thinks she has malaria or any illness. Even though she has had to wait and has been denied treatment, she explains that her only deterrent is financial.

From personal experience, Auma strongly believes that women should be legally entitled to inherit their husband's property/estate. She explains that she wishes she were a man, and that, if so, "I would be educated; and if I was not educated, I would be a farmer—a very good farmer. Also, I would not be an alcoholic; I would have one wife and few children; we would be happy."

Achieng'

At age 48, Achieng' is concerned about the changing social norms in her community. Achieng' has some tertiary education and 9 dependents, including children, nieces, nephews, grandchildren, and one neighbor's child. She says that when she observes young children these days, it is different from when she was raising her own. Achieng' thinks that girls and boys are born the same, that it is easy to raise them, but most of them are sexually active when they are very young. She is part of the Mother's Union, a group affiliated with the Anglican Church, and bases her decisions on biblical teaching and what her priest preaches. When discussing the relationship between husband and wife, Achieng' relied on the Bible, asserting that women and men cannot be equal. She quoted a section of the Bible that governs her marriage. In her opinion, a husband is the head of the home, and he guides and teaches his wife and children.

Achieng' is concerned about the amount of *chang'aa* being brewed and consumed in the community. If she were a village elder, she would ban *chang'aa.* In considering what her life would look like if she were a man, Achieng' said, "I would not be a drunk and not waste my money on alcohol, because it is often the case that women don't see the family income. Sometimes he leaves change with the bartender [laughs]; sometimes the money falls in the latrine and can't be retrieved." Achieng' has access to healthcare at the clinic, where her experiences have been good. She is particularly happy with the treatment she has received from one of the nurses there; they are members of the same church. Medication has always been available when Achieng' has visited the clinic, and although she has never used their (HIV, tuberculosis, or malaria) testing services, she is aware of their availability.

When discussing the family unit, Achieng' believes that it is acceptable—and inevitable—that men have multiple wives. She believes that women who have multiple partners are "morally loose" and are not socially acceptable.

Awino

Over the past decade, Awino has been a frequent visitor to the clinic. Awino, who is 36 years old, has a tertiary education and used to have a job in the community. She explains that some things have improved, but others remain consistently bad. The clinic now has better testing equipment, more medical staff, and, more often than not, medication available for purchase. She has had negative experiences at the clinic, as described here, yet she continues to visit the health center, even though she knows that her medical records are unsafe and that she will not always receive good care. When I asked her why, she explained that she couldn't afford to travel to a more expensive clinic. When Awino was in labor with her youngest child, she visited the clinic and had a traumatic experience—an experience she believes left her unable to have other children.

As is the case with most births in this rural community, Awino received minimal antenatal care, having no visits to this particular clinic. She freely explained the treatment that she received when she arrived at the clinic:

> Upon arriving at the clinic, I was met by the guard as usual. I told him that I was willing to pay for admission but if he could let the nurse know I was in labor, maybe she could take the money and fill in the rest of the information later. He left me there standing and went to inform the nurse in the back area. When he returned, he informed me that the nurse was on her tea break and showed me a bench to sit on, as I waited for her. I asked him to inform the nurse that I was about to have the baby. He agreed, only to return a few minutes later and inform me that labor takes hours. As if I didn't already know that, following the birth of my five children. So I waited. I waited for close to an hour and then gave birth to my daughter. Right there on that cement verandah, I gave birth to my youngest child. Alone. A few minutes later, the askari (police officer present at most government facilities) called the nurse, who scolded me for not warning them that I was that far along; she left muttering and complaining that she now had to clean the verandah. I cleaned the verandah. I was never admitted, or helped, so I took my child and we went back home. My daughter is now 8.

Awino (2010) wants her children to be highly educated and to have options because poverty is what keeps her going back to the same subpar clinic.

STRUCTURAL INEQUALITY: FACTORS MEDIATING WOMEN'S EXPERIENCES AT THE HEALTH FACILITY

A rich, varied body of results about education and the use of technology (see Sanya 2012; Sanya and Odero 2017) overshadowed some of the more salient and profound concerns about experiences at the local health facility and women's knowledge about education. However, during all of the interviews, the cost of healthcare came up, often leading to discussions about traditional medicine, with the women mentioning when they used traditional healing methods and where they received counseling and help in a private setting.

They compared the privacy and the cost of the traditional healing methods, citing unsanitary facilities as a reason to visit traditional healers.

Several of the women noted having been subject to traumatic experiences at the hands of medical practitioners. The experiences were recounted in either an ambivalent tone or with a great sense of injustice. The women who had higher levels of education recounted these experiences as an accepted reality; they never expressed that this treatment was unjust. When I asked a follow-up question, the most common response was, "That is how it is here."

By contrast, women with less than 5 years of formal education consistently expressed anger, asked if I thought that the same was true for rich people or in private institutions, and one woman asked if I had experienced injustice at the hands of medical practitioners. These questions revealed that the women in the study with less formal education were unwilling to normalize the negative experiences they described.

In addition to negative psychological and physical encounters with healthcare workers, the women spoke of a lack of confidentiality and expressed concerns about confidentiality; they explained that some nurses discussed patient files in the waiting room, naming the actual patients. The women said that they only visited the health center when the situation was dire because of its high cost and lack of privacy. Four women spoke of a medical practitioner who often shared patient's files with people in the community. One participant explained the situation by saying, "There was a doctor who was sacked from the health center. He used to take patient's files to the bar and then he would show off about being a doctor; he discussed women's private parts [vaginas]." This breach in confidentiality, which led to the doctor's dismissal, was a reflection of the treatment that the community received from its health practitioners. All of the women who had their personal information disclosed spoke of a fear of community judgment, scrutiny, and shame. The women also spoke about the lack of attention and monitoring of patients; Awino's birth experience, described above, represents an especially egregious case.

Other women recounted the lack of privacy, verbal abuse, and public disclosures of patient information. One woman explained, "The nurses talk about our cases with people in the waiting room: one time a woman walked out and [a nurse] told me what was wrong with her." This divulging of another patient's information not only violates the patient whose information has been shared but also informs the listening party that she is vulnerable in that setting and that her personal information may be shared with others.

The women also reported unhygienic conditions and mistreatment during childbirth. Their accounts of abuse, neglect, and a lack of confidentiality are consistent with research conducted on violations of women's human rights in Kenyan health facilities (Center for Reproductive Rights and Federation of

Women Lawyers–Kenya 2007). In some cases, like that of Awino, women described being forbidden from entering the health center. But what was most striking was how Awino retold her horrific account with a great deal of ambivalence—an ambivalence and an acceptance of injustice prevalent among women with more than 5 years of education. In numerous instances, acts of injustice were told as facts, as unchangeable historical acts.

IMPLICATIONS OF RESULTS

The variance based on education reveals that society's social ills must be reformed before education can be used to empower and emancipate women. Following Durkheim, who argued that education "is only the image and reflection of society. It imitates and reproduces the latter . . . it does not create it" (Durkheim 1951, p. 372), this research raises questions about women's relationship to power and how education intercedes or interferes with women's resistance. For instance, in KDHS (Kenya National Bureau of Statistics [KNBS] and ICF Macro 2014), abstract statements—e.g., "Education is a key determinant of the lifestyle and status an individual enjoys in a society"; "Studies have consistently shown that educational attainment has a strong effect on health behaviors and attitudes"; "[E]ducation increases with wealth and define education as instruction without addressing education as more than an economic process"—fail to capture or address the kinds of results seen in this study. Not only the role of education and increased education, but also education as a determinant of future success, are assumed to be a net positive. Yet the reality is much more nuanced. KDHS (Kenya National Bureau of Statistics [KNBS] and ICF Macro 2015) stipulates that households make "decisions about health, education, and general welfare" as well as "the source of drinking water; type of sanitation facility; building characteristics such as type of material used for the roofing, flooring, and walls; and number of rooms used for sleeping." This displaces formal education as the only factor that determines "future success." The factors that determine future success are more clearly understood in the embodied realities of women's lives—for instance, a comparison between Auma and Awino sheds light on the role that education plays in situ.

Auma is a widow with less than 5 years of education who is well respected in the community and has great leadership potential. She has experienced injustice in the limitations she has for decision making, access to power, and life choices; she also has limited access to financial resources. Auma not only shows an awareness of these limitations, she considers them unjust, wants different options available to her, and sees the gender disparity inherent in them. Awino, on the other hand, has more than 12 years of formal education, has previously participated in wage labor, and is aware of her options regarding better health care. Awino is systematically oppressed through both customary and national law but also through violence. She was silenced following her inhumane treatment at the hands of a health practitioner and, in her responses, appears to have accepted this injustice as something that she must live with—as a reality to be navigated, not resisted. Though both of these women are silenced in their public lives, Auma's and Awino's responses to marginalization are arguably shaped by their education levels. Auma, who has not been pacified through formal education, speaks about the injustice, while Awino accepts her treatment as an unchangeable reality in her life.

This juxtaposition of Auma and Awino poses questions about the role of education in silencing dissent and resistance. Does Awino's silence come from her institutionalized education? Considering the intimate historical connection between Kenya's formal educational system and colonialism and the role of education as a tool for civilization and oppression, Awino's responses show the "success" of education as a tool for pacification. The education system, inherited and maintained by the postcolonial government, is an important tool for maintaining both the political and economic agendas. Maintaining the need to foster quiescent and obedient subjects, the originally racially stratified education system was reappropriated, while the curriculum continued both to minimize African traditions and aspirations and to impose Western norms and values. Through a fusing of colonial education and indigenous values, formal education now seems to work toward normalizing discriminatory practices, as evidenced by Awino's description of her treatment at the clinic.

Auma, who is older than Awino, attended school during the colonial occupation and during Kenya's battle for independence. Four years of schooling didn't silence the indigenous education that she had. She benefited from an indigenous education that focused on training youth with survival skills and preparing them to assume certain responsibilities in the community. From my interview with Auma, it is evident that her knowledge of Luo folklore was not eroded by Western modes of thought. Contextualizing her experiences in history also suggests that she was named using traditional Luo practices, practices that assert personal responsibilities and social loyalties. In saying this, I do not argue that Auma's Luo sense of self remains intact, or that she remains unaffected by the patriarchy, colonialism, and capitalism around her. Rather, I suggest that regardless of the levels of erosion that may have occurred, Auma appears to conceptualize self-identity in indigenous Luo terms, as was the case before the introduction of formal Western education. Auma is perceived as a leader, she seeks leadership, and yet she can only envision this role if she were a man.

The results from my research raise the question, is education necessarily emancipatory? The results show that the shift from one culture to a significantly different one can sometimes create a trap in the hierarchy of one or both of those systems. It can limit the ways in which individuals navigate through certain social spaces and therefore stratify a society. This is not limited to women and certainly should not be ascribed to all cultural shifts. In the present case, however, education serves as a tool to support the system of social differentiation and stratification.

Education plays a vital role in regulating behavior and producing compliant citizens by teaching social norms and penalizing deviance. Most cultures already have indigenous forms of resistance and agency to appropriate and mediate life; these may overlap with universal movements, of course, but do not necessarily fulfill the same local function. For instance, although Luo culture suggests that land should be inherited by male relatives, when asked who should be legally entitled to inherit their husband's property/estate, all of the women interviewed asserted that widows should inherit land. This is a major resistance in this subsistence farming community given that women's land ownership and control have important connections with their empowerment; it defines social status and political power in local contexts, and it structures relationships both within and outside the household. Land is thus a productive asset that creates wealth and sustains livelihoods. Without secure access to land and a means of production—whether through traditional land inheritance or the women's proposed alternative of widow inheritance—the paradigm of daily survival compels the poor, due to circumstances beyond their control or influence, to live within short-term horizons that degrade resources and fuel a downward spiral of poverty. This shows that indigenous Luo resistance can, and still does, exist.

This resistance to Luo discrimination against women and its rejection of prevailing social hierarchies is slowly being eroded by formal education, the locus where Western-style stratification was inculcated into Luo society. Through the centralized, racialized, gendered, and ethnicized education system, existing social hierarchies are further reinforced while new hierarchies contingent on capitalist premises are solidified. Education in Kenya has become a tool that builds a subjugated subjectivity. To be emancipated, then, has transcended mere freedom from external (political) domination or aggression. If education is to provide emancipation and empowerment, it must be an innovative progression aimed not only at liberating and reenvisioning the self but also putting resources together for the betterment of the immediate society. As it is, emancipation and empowerment are located within the sphere of education through gestures like the push for entry into wage labor or through microcredit as forms of financial empowerment or entrepreneurship. These systems are hegemonic and define empowerment in neoliberal terms as well, such that colonial tools continue to reproduce subjugation through education. As such—no longer counterintuitively—the higher the level of education and the more embedded in their cultures, the more likely individuals will cling to existing structures of inequality that are normalized during processes of learning. Or, as the women in this study reveal: education functions as a normalizing force that maintains national ideologies and the status quo.

CONCLUSION

As an outgrowth of colonial civilizing and westernizing schools, education in Kenya valorizes, prioritizes, sometimes unquestioningly privileges, and typically entrenches Western innovation and international developments on health, sanitation, and water distribution as sites of advancement. Foregrounding the perils of an assumption that education is always directly linked to schooling and that either is necessarily emancipatory, this chapter has explored the lingering and new social effects of neocolonial hierarchies and imperialism on the lives of rural women in Kenya. In particular, education serves as a tool for social control, producing patriarchal subjectivities and normalizing inequity throughout the school system.

Women's gendered subjectivities are the product of social encounters, experiences, and relationships. These subjectivities are embodied in the norms and values that they ascribe to, that are imposed upon, and that they inhabit in order to live, thrive, and survive. Although formal education has the potential to foster inclusive gender patterns for all identities through curricula, this is not currently addressed in prevailing curricula. Merely to expose people to schools and education will not rearrange structures to disrupt the prevailing social norms defining lived experiences. Although each community has sites of governance, restriction, and resistance, these mechanisms now function in conjunction and in confluence with colonial-influenced education and ethnonationalist practices, as well as widespread patriarchal norms, thus intensifying the gendered limitations for accessing social services and public goods for women.

Chapter Four

Access to Safe Water, Women's Empowerment, and Decentralization Systems in Tanzania

Teresia R. Olemako

Efforts to access water, sanitation, and hygiene (WASH) are among key public health issues in developing countries such as Tanzania and are addressed in Sustainable Development Goal (SDG) number 6 concerning clean water and sanitation; namely to ensure availability and sustainable management of water and sanitation for all. Access to improved WASH facilities can promote socioeconomic development, reduce poverty, and alleviate burdens to women and children. According to Wasonga, Okawa, and Kiowi (2016) women and children play a major role in water household management, and any development interventions should consider women and children as key targets in the process. Safe water, sanitation, and hygiene practices are paramount to reduce morbidity and mortality rates among children (Wasonga, Okawa, and Kiowi 2016). In addition, access to safe water is a critical component in advancing the human rights of women (Brown 2010), as a disproportionate burden is placed on women in places where governments fail to provide sufficient water services (because where services are insufficient, women must walk long distances to fetch water for drinking, cleaning, and cooking). Women are active contributors in demanding implementation of human rights obligations. Women's engagement in decision making should be meaningful and create conditions in which women are able to question development processes in water management. For example, the World Bank (2012) cited India as a case study demonstrating that empowering women at the local level as economic, political and social actors changed the policy choices dramatically, and led to increases in the provision of water and sanitation services which marked significant achievement in improving lives of women and children. This chapter investigates gender roles and differential access to water resources as key factors in reducing gender gaps in Pangani river basin, Tanzania. A comparative research design allows me to consider livelihood niches and examine 360 households. I examine decentralization systems in Tanzania as an approach to water resource governance and their effect on water scarcity and the gender gap.

Tanzania Development Vision 2025, adopted in 2000, advocates for citizens of Tanzania to attain a high quality of life. Universal access to safe water and reduction of poverty are among necessary aspects embedded in quality of life. The United Republic of Tanzania (URT) recognizes the right to water and sanitation in line with the 2010 United Nations (UN) Resolution on the Right to Water and Sanitation (United Nations Office of the High Commissioner for Human Rights, United Nations Human Settlements Programme [UM-Habitat], and the World Health Organization 2010). Tanzania is among countries in East Africa supported by the United Nations and World Health Organization (WHO) in implementing WASH projects towards investing in and increasing access to water and sanitation, and reducing inequalities. Tanzania lacks the capacity to meet its water and urban sanitation Millennium Development Goal (The UN Water Global Analysis and Assessment of Sanitation and Drinking Water [GLAAS] Report 2014). So global aid commitments for water and sanitation were targeted to countries that needed financial support the most. In fact, sanitation and drinking water financial support "targeted to eastern and western Africa subregions increased from 43% to 65% (of total global aid commitments) . . . from 2008 to 2012" (WHO/UNICEF Joint Monitoring Programme for Water Supply and Sanitation 2015, p. 16). Despite external support, Tanzania is still facing challenges of water scarcity, and Water Point Mapping Tanzania national mapping shows 38% of 74,331 water points are not functional; whereas 7% are functional but need repair. Further, Taylor (2009) reported that 7.5% of rural Tanzanians lack access to clean and safe water due to functionality problems. Also, a survey of 55 out of 132 districts in Tanzania indicated that 43% of the water points were no longer working, and 25% of the water schemes had become nonfunctional within two years of installation. The situation has created water scarcity and has widened gender gaps because women are required to walk long distances searching for water. It is estimated that the average distance that women in Africa walk to collect water is 6 kilometers (3.7 miles). The Demographic and Health Survey Malaria Indicator Survey 2015–2016 Report (Ministry of Health, Community Development, Gender, Elderly and Children; Ministry of Health; National Bureau of Statistics; Office of the Chief Government Statistician; and ICF 2016) provides details for Tanzania:

> Fetching drinking water is an additional chore that could be of great cost to household members, depending on the time spent to obtain it. Four in 10 households (40%) spend 30 minutes or longer (round trip) to fetch drinking water; the figure is 52% in rural Tanzania Mainland, compared with 19% in urban

Tanzania Mainland and 14% in Zanzibar. [Ministry of Health, Community Development, Gender, Elderly and Children (MoHCDGEC) [Tanzania Mainland]; Ministry of Health (MoH) [Zanzibar]; National Bureau of Statistics (NBS); Office of the Chief Government Statistician (OCGS); and ICF 2016, p. 22].

The scenario of water scarcity and functionality problems highlight challenges faced by the river basin management system for water resources allocation in Tanzania, where water is perceived as an economic good, and therefore an important driver for economic development. The river basin management system created new problems, in contrast to the decentralized water resources allocation systems previously used in Tanzania, where water was perceived as a public good.

CHALLENGES OF THE RIVER BASIN MODEL AND DECENTRALIZED SYSTEMS

According to United Republic of Tanzania (2002a), when the river basin management system was introduced, water was newly allocated based on hydrological boundaries. As noted by the World Bank (2004), water scarcity in Tanzania became a national issue in early 1990, and administration of water resources via the river basin management system was meant to address the situation. After 1990, management of water resources in Tanzania was entirely based on the nine river basins that do not follow administrative boundaries as defined under the system of decentralized political structures (see Appendix 1). Under the river basin management structure, water is perceived as an economic good, while under decentralized systems, water is perceived as a public good. The river basin model practiced in Pangani town, the source of the Pangani River, is basically rooted in integrated water resource management (IWRM) and is perceived as being separate from the country's decentralized systems due to the presence of multiple actors from donor funding agencies in policy- and decision-making processes regarding water and land resources. The river basin model is a global model that was exported to several countries and, as reported by Hoag (2006), focused on industrial development, agricultural growth, and hydroelectric power generation but ignored social development. Donor agencies influenced how funding and expertise were provided and decided the types of technology employed and the projects to be undertaken. The construction of large dams was central to the river basin model to promote the intensification of agricultural production, electricity generation, and flood control. Lein and Tagseth (2009) presented three approaches to water governance in Pangani—state-centered, market-based, and community-based—and highlighted the problem of arriving at a single focus for development due to the use of the different development ideologies advocated by different professions. As Biswas (2008) contends, IWRM has not been "a universal solution" in terms of its results or application and is highly unlikely to deliver promising results in the future. Moreover, Lein (2004) questioned the practical applicability of a river basin management model given the relevant political and administrative boundaries. Lein (2004) quoted Barham's (2001) conclusion that the adoption of this model will definitively lead to conflict with democratic rights. Additionally, Kemper, Blomquist, and Dinar (2007) commented on the difficulties in integrating and decentralizing river basin management into the administrative system of a given country and highlighted the impact of time on achieving significant results. For example, authors noted that nearly a century was required before the benefits of integration were demonstrated in the Murray-Darling basin in Australia.

This chapter presents the case study of Pangani River basin in Tanzania and highlights that water scarcity faced in the country is deeply rooted in the governance system of the river basin water management model and decentralization systems. In this chapter I argue that addressing gender gaps is fundamental for women's empowerment, and this includes promoting better access to safe water, sanitation, and hygiene. This study builds on the African feminist framework (Zerai 2014) that argues that safe water, sanitation, and child health cannot be understood unless the socioeconomic, political, and cultural contexts are taken into account.

WHY DOES GENDER EQUALITY MATTER IN WASH?

Recent efforts concerning decentralization have focused on the decentralization by devolution (D-by-D) principle, with the aim of transferring power, functions, and resources to regions and local governments and thus providing equal opportunities for men and women to participate in development activities that affect their livelihoods. However, decentralization has failed to address gender gaps with respect to access to and control of productive resources such as water, sanitation, and hygiene (WASH). The major sources of this problem include inadequate institutional capacity, limited financial resources, and unclear roles and responsibilities for the central, regional, and local governments (due to, for example, the lack of a direct political link between central government ministries, departments, and agencies), which weakens the decentralization process and efforts to address gender inequalities across different dimensions. In the process, water scarcity is created, and poverty is experienced more severely by women than men due to biological and sociocultural vulnerabilities. Addressing gender equality is justified as fundamental in the Tanzania National Development Vision 2025, the MKUKUTA, and the National Strategy for Gender and Development (United Republic of Tanzania 2002b), all of which consider access to and control of productive resources to be of paramount importance to attaining sustainable livelihoods and a gender-inclusive society.

METHODOLOGY

The study was conducted in the Pangani River basin in Tanzania, which currently faces declining water flow amid competing needs and interests over water-resource utilization. A comparative research design across upstream, midstream, and downstream users was employed. The aim of this design was to compare three livelihood niches to seek an explanation for the similarities and differences in gender equality and to gain a deeper understanding of social reality in different contexts. As elaborated by Bryman (2004), the key factor to comparative design is the ability to distinguish the characteristics of two or more cases that may act as a supporting base for theoretical reflections on the contrasting findings. The comparative design utilizes both quantitative and qualitative research to present a better understanding of social phenomena. Multistage cluster sampling was employed because the population of the Pangani River basin is widely dispersed in four regions. As illustrated by Bryman (2004), cluster sampling is appropriate and reliable in terms of time and cost savings when dealing with a widely dispersed population such as that of the river basin under study.

The primary sampling unit was the Kilimanjaro region, due to its high percentage of household population (39.3% out of 574,907 total households) relative to the other three regions (see Appendix 2). The secondary sampling unit consisted of three wetlands and six villages identified around each wetland, out of which two villages were chosen per wetland. The selection was based on purposive sampling designed to capture differential livelihoods and attach gender attributes as they changed according to the gradient from upstream to midstream to downstream locations. The sampling was as follows: upstream (Lower Moshi irrigation scheme [LMIS]—Mabogini and Chekereni villages) paddy/rice plantations with rice as the wetland crop and the remainder as perennial crops such as maize, beans, and vegetables; midstream (Mawalla irrigation scheme [MIS]—Oria and Mawalla villages) paddy/rice cultivation and pastoralism; and downstream (Nyumba ya Mungu [NYM] dam—Lang'ata bora and Kiti cha mungu villages) with hydropower production, fisheries, and a dry season refuge for pastoralists from neighboring regions. The LMIS and MIS are both located in the Moshi rural district, while the NYM dam is in the Mwanga district. The selection of households, based on a participatory rural appraisal (PRA) survey from focus group discussion, time-series analysis, and transect walks was conducted in both NYM villages and identified three livelihood niches: irrigated agriculture, agro-pastoralism and fisheries that acted as a sampling frame for a stratified random sampling. In each livelihood group (i.e., niche), 120 respondents were selected, which entailed a total of 360 households for the whole study.

The sampling strategy was designed to capture gender relations among men and women performing differential livelihood options directly from wetland resources. Using a statistical formula by Yamane (1967) with a 95% confidence level and 0.05 precision, the sample of 360 respondents was established. The sample was considered adequate for the study, as according to Hair et al. (2006), any sample size usually suffices for descriptive statistics and is therefore considered suitable for rigorous statistical analyses. Sudman (1976) commented that if comparative analysis is to be performed between or within groups, a minimum number of 100 elements is needed for each group. Our sample meets this criterion.

The corresponding equation for a statistical formula for a selected sample is demonstrated here:

$$n = \frac{N}{1 + N(e)^2}$$

Where n = the sample size
N = the population size (total number of households)
e = the level of precision

Primary sources came from our own field survey and secondary sources (e.g., scientific journals, websites, official documents, reports, and books) from 2010 to late 2011. The research study employed a combination of qualitative and quantitative methods (Kanbur 2001; White 2002; Ellis and Mdoe 2003). Qualitative methods were used to address the policy and institutional context for multisector gender strategies, civil society organizations (CSOs), water, land and finance policies, decentralization, and governance levels. Quantitative methods were used to address gender-disaggregated data on household income, land holdings, credit schemes, education, savings, and investments.

A semistructured questionnaire was administered at the household level to the 360 respondents. The questionnaire was designed to provide useful information regarding household demographics (e.g., age, gender, marital status, household size, education, head of household), asset endowments, livelihood capital (e.g., natural, social, human, financial), gender roles, main livelihood options, and contributions to household economies. Data collected from the PRA and physical field visits are mainly qualitative in nature, and qualitative data analysis was used. Data from the semistructured questionnaire were analyzed using descriptive statistics (e.g., frequencies, mean, percentage of variables, and cross tabulation–chi square). Descriptive statistics were derived from the Statistical Package for Social Science (SPSS) for Windows, version 14.0. Questionnaire variable analysis was conducted with the procedure described in Pallant (2003).

DISCUSSION

Central Government: Budget Constraints

To complement efforts of global financial support in providing safe WASH facilities, the central government should demonstrate its commitment through setting sufficient budget lines to facilitate maintenance and sustainability of WASH projects and systems. The central government, as the highest level within the political structure, has a significant role in strengthening governance among sector ministries. As a state, however, it is considered weak in capacity, since approximately 50% of the budget is funded by external donors (United Republic of Tanzania 2010). The central government under the Ministry of Finance has a key role to strengthen governance when it comes to budget allocation among sectors, including water. Public expenditure review (PER) under the medium-term expenditure framework (MTEF) cross-sector strategy is used to prioritize sector requirements according to Poverty Reduction Strategy Paper (PRSP) objectives. However, as noted by United Republic of Tanzania (2009), "There is a problem of integrating water sector resource requirements from regions and local government authorities into the Ministry's input of the water sector to the budget guidelines." From year 2004–2005 to 2008–2009, the budget allocated for water sector has ranged from 309.1 to 397.6 billion Tanzanian shillings (Tshs), the equivalent of 3% to 5% of the total budget, and it ranks the least in priority compared to other sectors (Figure 4.1).

Trend analysis on the country's budget, specifically revenue and expenditures from year 2004–2005 to 2008–2009 as shown in Table 4.1, indicates the trend has been more or less the same, with minor slight changes especially in year 2008–2009. The percentage ratio for domestic revenue from total revenue in year 2004–2005 ranks 52% while donor contributions in the form of loans

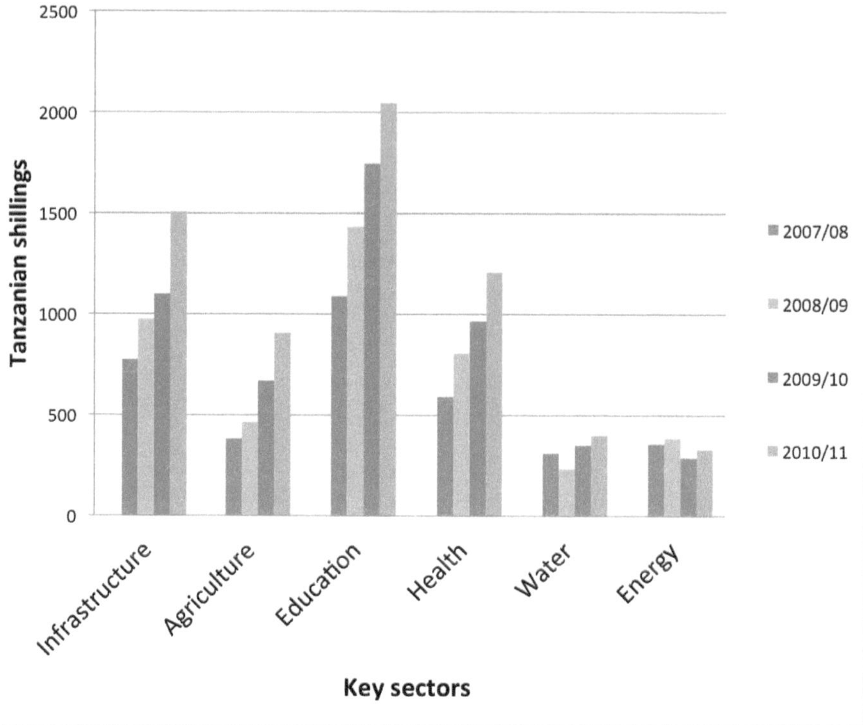

Figure 4.1. Budget Allocation among Sectors in Tanzania

Table 4.1. Budget for United Republic of Tanzania from 2004–2005 to 2008–2009 (in Millions of Tanzanian Shillings)

	2004–2005	*2005–2006*	*2006–2007*	*2007–2008*	*2008–2009*
Total revenue	**3,364,730**	**4,131,946**	**4,504,371**	**5,269,042**	**7,055,811**
Domestic revenue	1,733,709	2,124,844	2,739,022	3,634,581	4,240,074
LGAs' own source*	Nil	Nil	Nil	Nil	Nil
Foreign loans and grants	1,460,687	1,635,968	1,699,706	2,348,203	2,228,764
Borrowing	0	261,436	65,644	–713,742	541,973
Privatization proceeds	0	33,309	0	0	45,000
Total expenditures	**3,364,730**	**4,131,946**	**4,504,371**	**5,269,042**	**7,055,811**
Recurrent expenditures	2,124,580	2,788,580	3,167,160	3,458,070	4,925,442
Development expenditures	1,240,150	1,343,366	1,337,211	1,810,972	2,130,368
Local sources of funds	239,651	296,100	503,291	567,421	906,023
Foreign sources of funds	1,000,499	1,047,266	833,920	1,243,551	1,224,345

* LGA = local government authority.
Source: United Republic of Tanzania 2010.

and grants was 43%. In year 2008–2009, the percentage ratio for domestic revenue was 60%, while that of donors ranked 32%. There was a slight improvement in domestic revenue generation in year 2008–2009; however, it is important to note how revenue generated is spent in recurrent and development expenditures. Year 2004–2005 indicates 63% was spent in recurrent expenditures, while 37% was allocated to development projects. Of this 37% for development projects, 19% came from local sources and 81% from donor funding. Likewise, in year 2008–2009, the percentage ratio for recurrent expenditure was 70%, while development expenditures were 30%. Of the 30% for development projects, 42% came from local sources and 57% from donor funding. This scenario indicates more revenue is spent on recurrent expenditures (more than 50%), and less is allocated to development projects. Dependence on donor funding for development projects is highly pronounced, and this attitude is blocking innovation from local as well as central government to design mechanisms on how to tap potential revenues from sector ministries, including water and land resources. Table 4.1 indicates that nothing substantial is collected from local government authorities, the result of poor collection and unsystematic recording. Difficulty in collecting property tax on land is the major source contributing to poor revenues for local government authorities. Further, they have never considered water as a potential source of revenue.

Institutions Governing Water Resources

Water resources in Tanzania are being managed by the Ministry of Water under the Water Resources Management Act (United Republic of Tanzania 2009), Water Utilization (Control and Regulation) Act No. 42 of 1974 as amended by Act No. 10 of 1981 (United Republic of Tanzania 1981), Act No. 17 of 1989, Water Laws (Miscellaneous Amendments) Act No. 8 of 1997 and Water Laws (Miscellaneous Amendments) Act of 1999, which relate to the administration of granting of rights to water users. The regulations provide in detail for the granting of water rights (which began in 1975) and determine water use fees for various water uses. Traditionally water has been viewed as free resource (open access), a gift from God. The common property regime was the system used to manage water resources in the Pangani River basin. This was functioning under a traditional governance system until a water user rights system was reintroduced in 1990. The institutional setup for managing water resources in Tanzania falls under five main levels: from national level, basin level, catchment level, and district level to community level (i.e., water user associations).

According to United Republic of Tanzania (2002a), challenges facing water-resource management are that the existing approach is sector oriented, and it does not take into account multisectoral linkages in planning and budgeting the utilization and development of water resources. According to the National Water Sector Development Strategy (United Republic of Tanzania 2008), the functions of the Pangani Water Basin Office and all other basins' offices are to collect, process, and analyze data and coordinate water resource management; to issue, enforce, and revoke water rights and discharge permits and cooperate between sectors at the local level. However, research findings reveal that cooperation between sectors is missing since water resource planning is fragmented and is more sectoral, regional, and district oriented. A major reason for this is financial and human limitations to monitor about more than 2,500 abstractions in the river basin. As required by the Water Resources Management Act (United Republic of Tanzania 2009), monitoring whether water is put into beneficial use is not fulfilled. Research observations from the field noted the loss of water through poor irrigation methods and poor infrastructures in urban and rural water supplies as well as dormant water rights, which were counted as a source of revenue while the status is unknown. Linkages between land and water rights and between rules and modalities of operation are missing. Land is key when it comes to water-resource utilization. The need to merge institutional frameworks governing water and land resources by merging land rights and water rights is fundamental. Since the gap exists between water and land use investments, it is difficult to evaluate to what extent primitive accumulation of wealth and capital has occurred from utilizing water resources, while budget for the water sector is limited. In regards to development budgets, technology for water abstraction, storage, and reservoirs is highly needed.

Public Services and Basic Needs

Following the local government reforms program (1998–2008), the decentralization process has been designed to reduce the power of central authorities and to promote local autonomy at the lower levels. Decentralized public services have been poorly provided to the community since the implementation of the Structural Adjustment Policies (SAPs) in the 1980s. This circumstance is also partly due to the current budgetary constraints facing the financial sector in Tanzania. The reduction of public expenditures and the privatization of state enterprises to ensure a competitive economy were among the policy instruments implemented under the SAPs as the result of neoliberal economic policies and globalization. Reduced spending on major public services has contributed to the uneven ground between men and women in access to and control of productive resources, such as natural capital (e.g., land and water), human capital (e.g., education, skills, and knowledge), and financial capital (e.g., cash, credits, and liquefiable assets), as revenues generated from private activity are used to pay for public services and basic needs (i.e., a cost-sharing system), such as education, electricity, water, shelter, and fuel energy.

Descriptive data provide a sense of the types of housing in the Kilimanjaro region under study in 2010–2011, and access of those types to energy for household cooking, water, sanitation, and hygiene. Findings from the field survey (Figure 4.2) present household sizes by occupations, which vary considerably. A vast majority, 93.4% of workers in irrigated agriculture (n = 120) and 97.5% of workers in fisheries (n = 120), lived in households composed of one family (father, mother, and children). Household size for agro-pastoralists (n = 120) ranges from one family (16.7%) to two families (37.5%), three families (27.5%) and four families (18.3%), under the same compound sharing the same resources, which implies that women take on greater burdens with respect to domestic chores in agro-pastoralist households than in irrigated agriculture or fishery households.

Furthermore, food consumption per day is greater for agro-pastoralist household members than for other livelihood niches. Standards for shelter vary by occupation of the household head and are mostly shaped by differential access to building materials, affordability, and the nature of livelihood activities associated with family culture. Iron sheets (i.e., roofing materials) continue to dominate in most houses: 95% in irrigated agriculture households, 97.5% in fishery households, and 54.17% in agro-pastoralist households. Agro-pastoralists ranked last, with some houses still using thatching grass

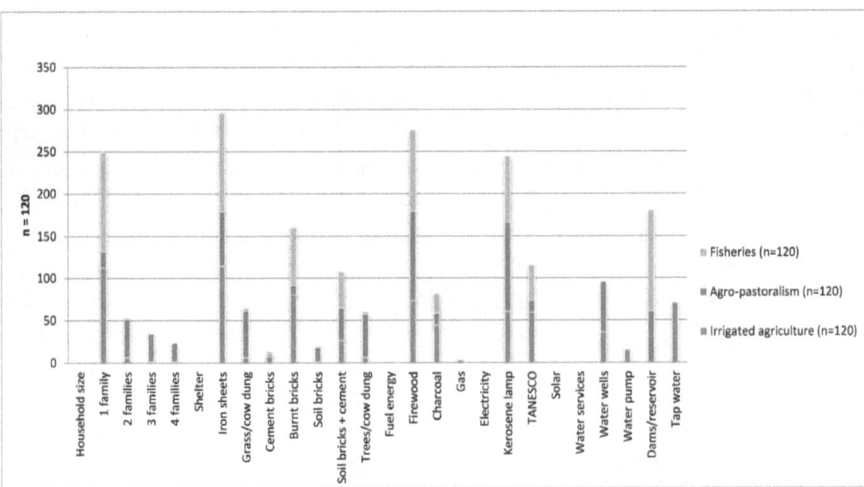

Figure 4.2. Public Services and Basic Needs in Kilimanjaro Region, 2010–2011 (Whole Sample)

and cow dung, which are easy to afford. Burnt bricks are popular construction materials highly used by small-scale farmers: 66.7% in irrigated agriculture households, 57.5% in fishery households, and 9.2% in agro-pastoralist households. Soil bricks plastered with cement are another material used to upgrade houses; wide use was noted by 21.7% of irrigated agriculture households, 35.8% of fishery households, and 31.6% of agro-pastoralist households. Pit latrines are also widely used by 58.3% of irrigated agriculture households, 92.5% of agropastoralist households, and 83.3% of fishery households. Squat toilets are also widely used by irrigated agriculture households (32.5%), fishers (11.7%), and agro-pastoralists (7.5%). (See Figure 4.2.)

Firewood remains one of the most important reliable sources of energy that is easily accessible and affordable for cooking, drying fish, and lighting by all livelihood niches: 60.8% of irrigated agriculture households, 80% of fishers, and 83.3% of agro-pastoralists. Charcoal is used to complement firewood in 36.7% of irrigated agriculture households, 19.17% of fishers, and 11.7% of agro-pastoralists. Other sources of fuel energy, such as gas and electric cookers, are not common due to low availability and affordability. The workload for women in collecting firewood still blocks efforts to reduce poverty in terms of time that could be spent in productive work. Further, forest degradation is noted mostly in the Mawalla Irrigation Scheme and the Nyumba ya Mungu gandazation dam, which has resulted in the siltation of the dam, especially during the wet season (Figure 4.2).

Electricity remains a problem in Tanzania. According to Reuters (2011), power rationing in the country was declared a national disaster after a prolonged drought and reduced water levels in 2011 following a deficit of 233MW, which is equivalent to 33% of the total net produced 700MW. Further, one-fifth of all generated electricity is wasted during transmission and distribution due to wear and tear on transmission equipment. Findings from the field survey on access to electricity supplied by the Tanzania Electric Supplies Company (TANESCO) indicate that upstream and midstream small-scale farmers in irrigated agriculture are better off in terms of electricity access (49.17% have access) than downstream fishers and agro-pastoralists, who do worse with access of 35% and 11.7%, respectively. Kerosene lamps are commonly used and easily accessible, but they have become expensive due to rising oil prices. The price for one liter of kerosene is equivalent to almost 2 USD, and large families can consume up to 2 liters per day. The figures for kerosene lamp usage were as follows: irrigated agriculture, 50%; fisheries, 65%; and agro-pastoralists, 83.3%. Use of solar power is not popular due to affordability constraints (Figure 4.2).

Access to domestic uses of water is still a major problem facing a majority of respondents in the study area (Figure 4.2). Upstream users in irrigated agriculture enjoyed the highest availability of tap water (58.3%), water wells

(29.2%), and water pumps (12.5%), while fishers depend entirely on fetching water directly from the NYM hydroelectric dam (100%). Approximately 50% of agro-pastoralists fetch water from the NYM dam, while the other 50% use water wells. Women in the fishing community spent a lot of time fetching water from the NYM dam. This circumstance contributed to poor hygiene, as the dam is used for fisheries, watering livestock, and domestic uses. Outbreaks of cholera and bilharzia are common around the NYM dam, which implies greater health costs to the family and a greater burden on women to look after the sick people.

Three major observations come from the research. First, variation in budgets targeted to different regions, local governments, sectors, and departments is what creates inequality in regions and local government and, in the process, unequal provision of public services. Second, inequality of staff salaries between those working in the central, regional, and local governments and those working in ministries, departments, and agencies kills work morale in the first group, as the second group is highly paid and enjoys proper training programs with adequate facilities and good working conditions. Third, the civil society organizations are slow in focusing on conflict resolution and resource governance and in providing significant outcomes such as operationalized schools, hospitals, and social protection services. This has contributed to the poor provision of public services and basic needs, widening gender gaps.

Level of Education and Dependence on Family Labor

Dependence on family labor is highly dominant in the study area, with fishers and agro-pastoral communities ranked the highest in promoting child labor for fish processing and selling, looking after cattle, and fetching water. According to United Republic of Tanzania (2008), child labor is prevalent, with 1.2 million reported children laborers in 2000 and 2001. Child labor is evident in the study area and cited as the major source of labor in irrigation fields, grazing, and fishing sites. Among agro-pastoralists, children are quite often used as cattle herders. The study revealed that this practice is passed down from one generation to the next, limiting the young generation's access to formal education and the ability to diversify to other livelihood options. The results indicate that the correlation between education levels and dependence on family labor is highly significant ($p < 0.00$). The situation is worse for fishers and agro-pastoralists located midstream and downstream compared with irrigated agriculture located upstream. Percentage ratios indicate that out of 360 respondents, 71% with a primary-level education or below (i.e., no education) depend on family labor, out of which agro-pastoralists rank the highest (41%), followed by fishers (36%) and small-scale farmers in irrigated agriculture (23%). (See Figure 4.3.)

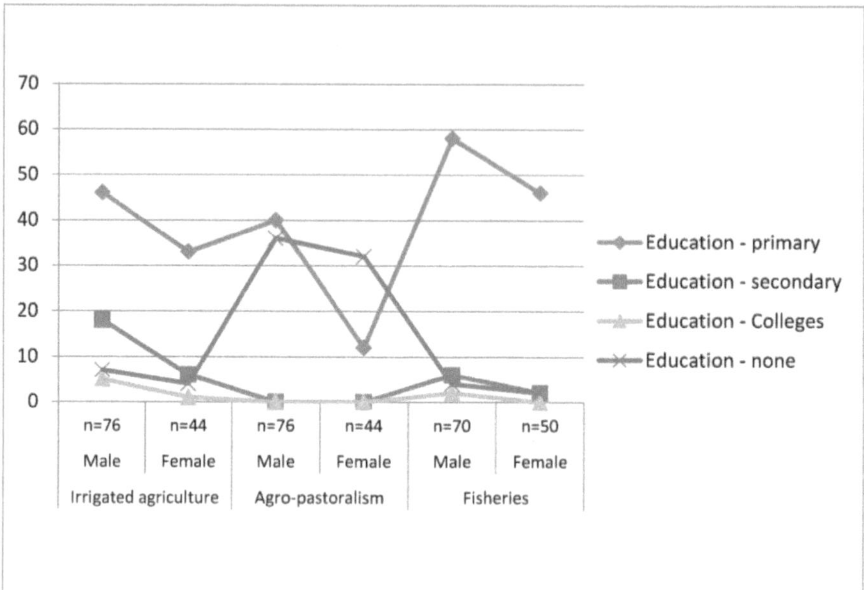

Figure 4.3. Respondents' Levels of Education in Survey of Tanzanians (Whole Sample)

Out of 120 respondents (males = 76; females = 44) in irrigated agriculture, 60.5% and 23.7% of males accessed primary school and secondary education, respectively, while 75% of females possessed a primary school education and 13.6% advanced to secondary school. In the agro-pastoralist community, 52.6% of males accessed primary school education, with 0% attending secondary school and 47.4% having never been to school/not knowing how to read and write, while 27.3% of females accessed primary school education, with 0% attending secondary school and 72.3% not knowing know how to read and write. In the fishery community, 82.8% of males possessed a primary school education and 8.6% advanced to secondary school, while 92% of women had been to primary school and 4% to secondary school. As put forward by United Republic of Tanzania (2002b), both men and women are involved in reproductive, productive, and community roles. However, women in rural and urban areas are subjected to a heavy burden, as men restrict them from engaging in other productive work. Women in rural areas spend 16 to 18 hours per day working, including fetching water, while men work 8 to 10 hours per day. Traditions, culture, and low levels of education are the main causes of the unequal division of labor.

Chapter Five

Gender as Social Structure and Its Potential Impact on Safe Water and Sanitation Technologies in East Africa

An African Feminist Analysis

Assata Zerai and Rebecca L. Morrow

In this chapter, we assess safe water and sanitation technologies through the lens of African feminism. Specifically, we look at current and proposed projects of researchers who are a part of the Safe Global Water Network. Seeded by the Safe Global Water Institute (SGWI), the Safe Global Water Network

> is a consortium of global centers of excellence in research, education, and regional stakeholders working across the boundaries of Water & Sanitation with Health, Food, and Energy. United, we are working to overcome the basic science, engineering solutions, educational capacity, and socio-economic barriers to providing sustainable safe water and sanitation to the peoples of the world. (University of Illinois Board of Trustees 2017)

While most members of the Safe Global Water Network are engineers, we bring a social scientific sensibility and feminist approach to its work. Here, we examine gender as a social structure and its potential impact on safe water and sanitation technologies in East Africa.

Access to and the uptake, implementation, and acceptance of technological innovations is influenced by social context and a community's social structure. Aspects of the social structure to consider in East African contexts include gender, class status (including socioeconomic status, income, and education), religion, ethnicity, and residence in rural versus urban areas. Here we focus primarily on considering gender as social structure in the development and implementation of new water and sanitation technologies in states and in resource-insecure communities, such as the Kibera informal settlement of Nairobi in Kenya, which has low infrastructure relative to proximate better-resourced areas, and refugee settlements near Arusha, Tanzania, and Kampala, Uganda.

One of our overriding questions is this: How can development policy be instituted in a way that does not contribute to securing and reproducing structures and practices of inequality? There are lessons that can be learned from the experiences of citizens of African nations and refugees located there. These lessons may be adapted to communities that are looking to incorporate new safe water and sanitation technologies, but first consideration must be given to ways to implement these technologies without reproducing inequality. Clearly evidence of a democratic and nonrepressive political environment is a necessary condition for success. Even with the hard work and integrity of many citizens committed to social advancement, needed are health policy by which officials seek to redress the dearth of rural and periurban infrastructure and health resources; health policy, planning, and execution that is inclusive of input from health practitioners, activists, women, and marginalized members of society; and international support in forms that follow the lead of citizens and are based on best practices.

The political will to provide resources to citizens is another necessary condition for successful implementation of development policy. One example is the case of South Africa following the end of apartheid. After political independence in 1994 when the government was finally able to make strides in providing health resources to all citizens regardless of race, the AIDS epidemic ravaged many communities. This step back was due largely to the country's history of forced migrant labor during apartheid and the AIDS denialism of President Mbeki and the Ministry of Health, resulting in lack of attention to prevention and treatment efforts until 2010. Until 2010, the lack of political will severely undercut South Africa's nascent improvements in health care.

As shown in chapter 4, a program for equitable distribution of development resources, such as water and sanitation, can be only as strong as both the infrastructure in the region and the state's democratic process. However, examining the process of developing water and sanitation technologies is another crucial intervention. In the following pages, we (1) outline features of an African feminist analysis of new technologies that are acceptable and appropriate, (2) discuss the valiant efforts by researchers, health professionals, civil servants, donors, nongovernmental organizations, and others to increase access to safe water and adequate sanitation, (3) analyze each of these examples with a gender lens, and then (4) make suggestions for how policymakers, engineers, and other stakeholders might develop intervention strategies that will not exacerbate gender inequality.

WAYS TO UTILIZE AFRICAN FEMINIST METHODOLOGY TO ASSESS NEW TECHNOLOGIES

Upon reviewing "the role and contribution of feminism as a liberating paradigm within Africa's scholarly community between 1990 . . . and 2010"

(Mama 2011, p. 3), leading African feminist Professor Amina Mama states, "It is ethically indefensible to neglect gender" (2011, 19). Bringing gender front and center, we ask, How could better water and sanitation technologies contribute to gender equity and social justice and improve the lives of especially girls and women? And how do we describe the direct and indirect impact that sanitation can have on a woman in terms of quality of life for her and her family? As noted in this book's introduction, social justice advocacy describes efforts to increase fairness in the distribution of resources; end discrimination against all groups, fostering values that recognize all people as equal; and promote the participation of people in policy and implementation processes that affect their lives and promote transparency and accountability for how decisions are made and how they impact society (Klugman 2011).

Clearly, better access to improved water and sanitation contributes to social justice because it increases fairness in the distribution of this crucial resource to communities. In regard to gender equity, one way the lack of sanitation in African settings affects women is by making them vulnerable. For example, in Kenya's informal settlement of Kibera and other settlements including Mathare, Kariobangi, Kawagware, Kangemi, Mukuru-kwa-Njenga, Mukuru-kwayaba, and Dandora in Nairobi, sanitation facilities are woefully inadequate. As noted in other chapters, Amnesty International reports (2010) that it is common that pit latrines shared by more than 100 people are a 10-minute walk or more for most residents. This not only increases environmental contamination from improper alternative methods of disposing of human waste (Katukiza et al. 2010, p. 52)—but it adds to violence and insecurity of especially female residents and children. The lack of improved sanitation facilities is common in unplanned settlements. In Bwasie III near Kampala, for example, 75% of residents use shared toilets (Katukiza et al. 2010, p. 52). The safety concerns for women that arise when they do not have access to adequate toilet facilities on their premises is a concern in especially resource-insecure sites such as Kibera and in refugee settlements near Kampala, Uganda, and the Arusha region of Tanzania. In a World Bank report, authors note that "women who lack sanitation often risk sexual harassment on the way to and from their defecation site. . . . The emancipation that a latrine (on their premises) bestows on such women cannot lightly be dismissed" (Cairncross and Valdmanis 2006).

Lack of cleanliness is another risk to women. Tumwebaze and Mosler (2014) conducted a cross-sectional study of 424 household respondents living in three unplanned settlements near Kampala. The respondents were primarily using shared toilets, with about 100 users per toilet. Of the 41 toilets frequented by respondents, researchers found that 66% were unclean, with over half reported as "quite dirty, dirty, or very dirty" (p. 8). And women carried the lion's share of the burden of cleaning communal toilets. "Cleaning of the shared toilets was largely attributable to gender. More than two-thirds of the respondents (73.1%) reported that females were mainly responsible for the cleaning of shared toilets" (Tumwebaze and Mosler 2014, p. 8). So having shared toilets requires more work on the part of women.

If toilets are not cleaned regularly, diseases may spread. Another hazard of shared toilets is the impact of bacteria on health. In a study of 51 countries, Fuller et al. (2014) find that "shared sanitation appears to be a risk factor for diarrhea" (p. 173) among young children. Japheth Kwiringira and colleagues (2016) discuss the multiplicative effect of the wet season and shared toilets on health outcomes of unplanned settlement residents in Kampala. They argue that during "the wet season and when human activities are at their peak, sanitation is most dire in poor slum populations" (p. 361). Cholera outbreaks are more likely to occur in the wet season, as has been the case in Kampala city (Kwiringira et al. 2016, Legros et al. 2000). Unclean shared facilities spread pathogens. "Pathogens form a major cause of disease transmission due to their presence in human excreta and when mixed with wastewater, the pathogens flow downstream and spread in the environment especially during flooding (Kwiringira et al. 2016; Katukiza et al. 2010, p. 52; Feachem et al., 1983; Prüss et al., 2002; Niwagaba et al., 2009)" (Katukiza et al. 2010, p. 52; for details on references cited within the quote, see the source publication). Researchers conclude that "poor sanitation in slums is part of a broader urban mismanagement conundrum pointing towards the urgent need for multiple interventions aimed at improving the general urban living conditions well beyond sanitation" (Kwiringira et al. 2016, p. 1).

Netsayi Mudege and Eliya Zulu (2011) discuss the challenges of access to clean water for residents of unplanned settlements in Nairobi City. Results show that the problems concerning water provisioning within Nairobi slums are less about water scarcity and more about unequal distribution and the marginalization of slum areas in development plans. Though the Kenyan government has worked to provide improved sources of drinking water to the country's residents, including its most vulnerable by implementing the Pro-Poor Implementation Plan for Water Supply and Sanitation in 2007, many challenges abound. Some of these challenges, according to the *Analytical Report on Housing Conditions, Amenities and Household Assets* (Kenya National Bureau of Statistics 2012, p. 17), include the following:

- Cost of service: The poor pay 5 to 10 times more for water supply and sanitation (WSS) services than the rich who have ready access to services.
- Access to services: The urban and rural poor have limited access to WSS services.

- Attracting private investment capital: The funds available from the government and development partners are not enough to meet the Millenium Development Goals (MDGs) [and now Sustainable Development Goals].
- Corporate governance: It is difficult for stakeholders in the Water Service Boards (WSBs) and Water Service Providers (WSPs) to hold their directors and top managers to account.

Given that the poor pay not just more for water supply and sanitation, but *5 to 10 times more*, the pro-poor policy is found severely wanting. Mudege and Zulu (2011) explain that "poor water management, lack of equity-based policies and programmes, and other slum-specific features such as land-tenure systems and insecurity exacerbate water-supply problems within slum areas" (p. 221). Respondents in Mudege and Zulu's study relate that they are second-class citizens in Nairobi and that their needs fall behind those who have greater power and prestige. According to the United Nations (2010, p. 2),

> The water supply and sanitation facility for each person must be continuous and sufficient for personal and domestic uses. These uses ordinarily include drinking, personal sanitation, washing of clothes, food preparation and personal and household hygiene. According to the World Health Organization (WHO), between 50 and 100 litres of water per person per day are needed to ensure that most basic needs are met and few health concerns arise.

The basic human right to clean water is denied by the intermittent and insufficient access provided to residents of unplanned settlements in Nairobi. Multiple respondents in Mudege and Zulu's study indicate that during "profitable events like the Nairobi Agricultural Show" (2011, p. 227), water "supply is interrupted. Especially at the times of the Nairobi show . . . you know all the pipes [are] diverted to the show ground. At the time of the show we normally have a lot of water problems here" (p. 227).

In addition to intermittent access, a clear, indirect association between sanitation and education is likely, as poor sanitation affects the nutritional intake and health of children and adults alike (Griffiths 2013; Smith et al. 2013). Poor sanitation at school sites can contribute to school children's illnesses and the spread of disease. Further, as noted in an earlier chapter, safe sanitation in schools would likely increase the safety of girls in schools and improve health outcomes so that children miss fewer days of school. The long-term health outcomes of children would lead to lower stunting and wasting of children (Smith et al. 2013; Humphrey 2009) and better physical and mental development so that they can better retain what they learn in school. In this case, it would improve education of adults over the long run because the improved sanitation of children and their resulting improvements in education would likely improve life chances in the future when they become adults.

Water, Sanitation, and Quality of Life

Water and sanitation clearly can have an important impact on quality of life. According to the World Health Organization (2014),

> Quality of life benefits include time saved searching for and carrying water and using distant or unsafe facilities; improved school attendance and completion, especially for girls; fewer days lost in the home, at school or work due to preventable sickness; greater comfort, privacy and safety, especially for women, children, the elderly and people living with disabilities; a greater sense of dignity and well-being for all. Economic benefits include an overall estimated gain of 1.5% of global GDP and a US$ 4.3 return for every dollar invested in water and sanitation services due to reduced health care costs for individuals and society; greater productivity and involvement in the workplace through better access to facilities, especially for women in the workforce; opportunity for growth of new industries, such as infrastructure, disposal and use of human waste and materials supply. (p. 10)

Researchers from the Department of Civil and Environmental Engineering at the University of Illinois examined the impact of sanitation on quality of life and ways in which this can work through three nexuses: energy, health/nutrition, and fertilization. Regarding the energy nexus, the extraction of methane potentially increases energy production. The ability to cook is one of the benefits that have been identified. Implementation of technologies to make households self-sustaining clearly has multiple quality of life benefits. Regarding the health/nutrition nexus, Professor Jeffrey Griffiths and his group at Tufts University are doing cutting-edge work on environmental enteropathy and the improved health of children resulting from better sanitation in Uganda. We draw on this work in our discussion of sanitation and improved educational outcomes (as an indirect effect of sanitation). Sanitation and extracting nutrients from human and animal waste is the third nexus. Nutrient extraction may help to better fertilize soil and increase crop yields. Better crops (taken with improved sanitation and fewer environmental contaminants) mean higher quality nutritional intake for families. And better-fertilized crops could also mean farmers' commanding higher prices in the marketplace.

CURRENT EFFORTS TO PROVIDE SAFE WATER AND SANITATION ON THE AFRICAN CONTINENT

When creating and implementing safe water and sanitation technologies, we argue, a framework for understanding the impact on gender must be identified and every effort must be made to help eradicate these inequalities. Normally, when water and sanitation technologies are being assessed, analysts take "into account sustainability criteria, including social acceptance, technological and physical applicability, economical and institutional aspects, and the need to protect and promote human health and the environment," as in Katukiza et al. (2010, 52). But a framework that takes into account elements put forth by feminist researchers addresses issues such as social justice and centering women in project design and implementation, and these important values are central in sustainable implementation of water and sanitation technologies. We examine three such values here.

The first is this: "Identifying the subject of study in ways that ring true to women in the setting, so that their interests drive research agendas and research is African-centered and woman-centered" (Zerai 2014, p. 90). According to Imam, Mama, and Sow (1997), "engendering African social science is not a simple development of knowledge, but is also necessarily and simultaneously profoundly a political struggle over power and resources" (p. 2). They argue that "social science which does not acknowledge gender as an analytic category is an impoverished and distorted science, and cannot accurately explain social realities and hence cannot provide a way out of the present crisis in Africa" (p. 2). The necessity of scholar-activism and participatory action research has been elaborated elsewhere (Imam and Mama 1994; Mama 2000; Sudbury 1998; Collins 1990). For example, Ampofo et al. (2004) explain that "the notion that research methods and techniques are atheoretical has been challenged, as are the false ideas of scientific neutrality and the separation of politics, theory, and methods" (p. 687). Amina Mama, Iyesha Imam, and Fatou Sow explain, "Gender analysis, gender-aware analysis or gendered analysis may focus on women . . . but in a way that clearly recognizes the gender relations which construct historically its subject" (1997). Gender analysis can be applied and must be applied to all areas of inquiry. In *Engendering Social Science*, Imam, Mama, and Sow (1997) "challenge the androcentricity of social science knowledge by explaining how and through what mechanisms much of social science ignores and marginalizes the contribution that women make to society, and helps to inferiorize and subordinate women by generating sexist knowledge which legitimates the male-dominant social order" (p. 8). Further, Imam, Mama, and Sow (1997) argue the importance of Africa-centered analysis. "There is a concern not simply with understanding, but with producing a form of knowledge that can help to transform oppressive realities" (p. 26). In considering the importance of these issues stated by African feminist scholars, we operationalize this as "*interests of subjects drive research agenda.*"

The second value we address is *attention to the most marginalized members of society*. For example, Kwiringira and colleagues (2014) argue that studies analyzing "progressive improvements in sanitation . . . have not indicated barriers faced by the urban poor" (p. 624). As shown above, the urban poor, including those living in refugee and unplanned settlements, in many societies lack access to improved water sanitation (African Population and Health Research Center 2014). Further, this population is vast. Most of the growth in urban areas occurs in unplanned settlements. As of 2008, "about 71% of urban residents in Kenya live in slums" (Kyobutung et al. 2008, p. 1). In more recent data, "there are approximately 2.5 million slum dwellers in about 200 settlements in Nairobi representing 60% of the Nairobi population and occupying just 6% of the land. Kibera houses about 250,000 of these people. Kibera is the biggest slum in Africa and one of the biggest in the world" (African Population and Health Research Center 2014). "About 70 per cent of urban residents in most cities in Tanzania live in unplanned settlements, slums or squatter areas" (SADC/SARDC 2012, p. 102; UN-Habitat 2009). According to the World Bank (2015), "6.4 million Ugandans live in urban areas . . . and . . . at least 60 percent of the urban population in Uganda [are] living in slums" (p. 2). So though this concern addresses marginalized members, in urban contexts, especially, marginalized persons are not only numerous, but often the majority. We operationalize this as consideration of the impact on women, including the marginalized.

The third value is this: that women's agency is built on and enhanced through consulting with women and working with them to design new water and sanitation technologies with their lived realities in mind, and that the important cultural exigencies considered in implementation include consideration of the gender social structure of a community. The ABANTU women's research collective states relevant criteria for research that is people-centered, that is very relevant to technological interventions that are appropriate. They promote research "to empower African people to participate at local, national and international levels in making decisions which affect their lives, enabling action for change. . . . Women have a vital role to play in policy-formulation and public decision-making, yet there are few African women with the necessary education or experience to enable them to fulfill this role" (as quoted in Mama 2000, 60). There is a linkage between gender equality and equitable distribution of resources. Scientists, civil servants, NGOs, and other stakeholders involved must be *intentional* about incorporating women's voices in technological design and implementation. We operationalize this as women being consulted in the design and implementation of new water and sanitation technologies. Researchers, donors, and corporate actors who want to introduce new technologies, ostensibly to improve the lives of individuals, must consider the impact on women and children and must not consider their technology a success as long as it creates new inequality or exacerbates existing gender inequity.

ANALYSIS OF CURRENT EFFORTS USING A GENDER LENS

Members of the Safe Water Global Network (SWGN) presented their current projects at the 2013 Safe Global Water and Sanitation Institute Summit held in Arusha, Tanzania, January 28–30. (Select presentations are detailed in Table 5.1.) The purpose of the summit was to create a multidisciplinary and multi-institutional group to combine advances in development and academic research for creating innovative partnerships to solve issues of water and sanitation. The group is dedicated to finding revolutionary and global solutions, remembering that a one-size-fits-all solution is untenable.[1]

Presentations were grouped into three main categories: combining safe global water and sanitation with issues of health, environmental sustainability and energy, and nutrition and food. We outline here those projects to provide a sense of current work by researchers, industry, and water and sanitation governance specialists to enhance environmental sustainability and provide communities with adequate water and sanitation. As is evident from the project details, many researchers and others directly consult with women in their projects and/or consider the needs of and impact on women in their design. Others do not mention relevance of their work to women's lives.

Environmental Sustainability and Energy Nexus

Sanitation systems worldwide, when outdated, must be overhauled. This is not a concern limited only to the Global South; rather it is about ensuring that contemporary, continually deteriorating water and sanitation systems are improved by innovations to address concerns specific to a locale. In most places, the systems require tremendous amounts of water and upkeep and must have better resiliency in the face of extreme events. The failed infrastructure of sanitation systems also contributes to water's becoming toxic. A new paradigm must be created where new solutions are built that are tailored to individual communities and ensure that wastewater is used as a resource through harvesting fertilizer and recycling water. Partnerships must arise that focus on local and regional approaches (Drewes 2013). Scientists at the University of Illinois at Urbana-Champaign are creating systems that can convert wastewater into energy and water that can be reused. However, convincing people in the community that such water is safe will be problematic. Science and technology must adapt to the understanding of the culture. In order to be successful, projects must follow the three pillars of sustainability: social, economic, and environmental. All three must be examined before building to understand how the culture will affect the long-term sustainability of the project (Guest 2013). Dr. Peiying Hong of King Abdullah University of Science and Technology works to reduce microbial contaminants from reclaimed water.

Table 5.1. Select Presentations from the Safe Global Water and Sanitation Institute Summit, January 2013

Title	*Presenter Affiliation*	*Statement of Problem*	*Solution*	*Gender Consideration*
Clean Household Services: Building Energy and Water?	Tami C. Bond, University of Illinois at Urbana Champaign	The fourth leading cause of death in countries of the Global South is solid cooking fuels used in the house to prepare meals. Burning wood, coal, etc., produces waste products in the air and fire.	Technology must be created that will work in the field, with perhaps multiple uses, such as a cookstove that also pasteurizes water.	Women are consulted in design and implementation. Impact on women is considered.
Household Water Treatment for Prevention of Diarrhea Disease in Tanzania	Nesia Mahenge, PSI (Population Services International)	The goal is to provide distribution and promotion of quality water. With many dying of diarrhea and in support of the Millennium Development Goals, PSI seeks to promote healthy behavior to help prevent contamination. They provide safe drinking water targeted to women, pregnant women, caretakers, and those with AIDS and, secondarily, to provide health care for teachers and children.	Through pharmacies, PSI distributes free Waterguard nationally, including training for proper use. Targeted community activists train and distribute Waterguard to improve water for children under 5 and to encourage breastfeeding. The trainers train community members who use bicycles to continue teaching and distribution, as well as to measure if people are still using Waterguard.	Women are consulted in design and implementation. Impact on women is considered.
Community Ownership of Safe Water, Hygiene, and Sanitation Practice	Simon Kajala and Mika Ayo, OIKOS East Africa	Any time a solution is implemented in a community, we must consider the technical and social part. They focus on the social part to make sure that community ownership is in place and that the services are sustainable and equitably based both upstream and downstream.	This partnership between rural communities, women, school children (women and school children do the most walking to obtain water), and local community organizations use the water supply from a spring in Arusha National Park. The process empowers the community.	Women are consulted in design and implementation. Impact on women is considered.

HWTS Successes and Challenges in East Africa	Daniele Lantagne, Tufts University	There are five proven household options for water treatment that reduce diseases: ceramic filtration, chlorination SWS (safe water system), solar disinfection, bios and filtration, PuR. There is no one-size-fits-all solution to household water treatment solutions because of differing cultural views.	In Zambia, 42% of the population use chlorination successfully. However, due to a technological failure, in the Dominican Republic a biosand filter took clean water and made it unclean. SODIS will not work in cultures where hot water is seen as bad.	Women are consulted in design and implementation. Impact on women is considered.
The SWAP Program in Kenya: Using Local Community Members as Long-Term Change Agents	Alie Eleveld, SWAP (Safe Water and AIDS Progress)	This project distributed Waterguard and found that only 1% of the problems were technology; 99% were distribution. Publicity: user acceptability is slow when users cannot see immediate change. Sustainability: cost effective implementation of consumer demand. For distribution, SWAP used the local community to take care of residents' own health. They used social marketing and engaged the community through entrepreneurship, recruiting and training trainers.	Through community engagement, SWAP has created a baby and family care center that includes a community training and education center. Women have become empowered through business and children have received better health care. Perhaps this solution would find success in other rural locations.	Women are consulted in design and implementation. Impact on women is considered.

(continued)

Table 5.1. *(Continued)*

Title	*Presenter Affiliation*	*Statement of Problem*	*Solution*	*Gender Consideration*
Community Perspectives: Addressing Water Quality Challenges in the Bondo District	Odundo Rodriguesn and Bondo Wandiga, University and University of Nairobi	This group is finding better water treatment solutions for the Lake Victoria area.	A survey was conducted with 658 women and 852 men about how they obtained water. The jerry can causes illnesses and is an indication of poverty. Gender was not part of design, but no results were found.	Impact on women is considered.
Africa User Research in Water Sanitation	Jennifer Foster, ATH	In order for successful programs, we must find products that are affordable for those with low or no income.	We must work with end users to explore what is feasible in their communities, technology experts on the design, and then validate with end users.	Women are consulted in design and implementation. Impact on women is considered.
Using Bottom-Up Understanding to Design Solutions for Subsistence	Madhu Viswanathan, University of Illinois at Urbana Champaign	This research group is combining a micro-lending university partnership with an NGO. By using a bottom-up strategy, they are addressing poverty through the use of a market exchange. They are not using any macroeconomic structures.	The group teaches about market and then they design solutions. The community members are experts at surviving so the university members use that expertise realizing they have none in this area.	Women are consulted in design and implementation. Impact on women is considered.

Gender as Social Structure in East Africa and Its Potential Impact on Safe Water	Assata Zerai, University of Illinois at Urbana Champaign	All programs must be created without creating more inequality. It is imperative to create a baseline when entering communities to ensure that the social structures, especially gender, are understood.	Gender norms should not impede implementation. As groups enter communities, they must understand the culture and directly ask for ways that implementation might cause or exacerbate inequality. We must directly and systematically prevent exclusion as much as possible.	Women are consulted in design and implementation. Impact on women is considered.
Impact of Irrigation on Nutrition, Health and Gender Outcomes	Claudia Ringler, International Food Policy Research Institute	Irrigation is increasing in Africa. The way people are engaged greatly affects outcomes in nutrition, health, and gender. When women are more empowered, there are larger poverty-reducing impacts. Gender issues include water needs and preferences, shifts in production systems, and shifts in control.	When creating new systems or improving old ones, researchers must understand how irritation, nutrition, health and gender are related. Consider reuse and make sure unintended consequences are examined. For example, pesticides in India caused infertility.	Women are consulted in design and implementation. Impact on women is considered.
Producing Safe Food Where Irrigation Water Is Polluted: From Risk Assessment to Risk Mitigation	Phillip Amoah, International Water Management Institute	When irrigation water is polluted, we must consider the risks and benefits. The raw sewage causes severe water pollution and is a risk for consumers, farmers, local families, and a loss of life years to diarrhea. However, the benefit of fertilizer causes increased yield which supports many jobs and livelihood especially for women.	Urban farmers earn more than rural farmers and women earn more than men. It is important to reduce risk of E. coli from farm to market using the QRMA method. The risk can be reduced through a multiple barrier approach.	Women are consulted in design and implementation. Impact on women is considered.

Chlorination does not necessarily disable antibiotic-resistant viruses in fecal bacteria; engineers must also understand microbiology to create a membrane bioreactor to reduce bacteria and must gain an understanding of the effects on agriculture when the reclaimed water is used (Hong 2013).

Beyond sanitation issues, Professor Tami Bond creates a more sustainable solution to solid fuels in the home. Waste products in air and fire are the fourth most common cause of death. Like the sustainability issues mentioned above, a cultural paradigm must be created that will ease a transition to more sustainable cooktop solutions. Communities will perhaps be more accepting of a solution that helps ameliorate some of the competing issues of time, focus, and funding. Perhaps if a stove could cook and pasteurize water, acceptance would be easier. Bond also urges members of the network to ensure an end to the days of deploying technologies and then leaving. There are missed opportunities when networks are not maintained, especially when technology proves unsustainable, for whatever reason (Bond 2013).

In addition to university experts, SGWN consists of nongovernmental organizations and companies, which bring their expertise of producing technology and implementation to the fore. Dr. Sangam Tiwari (2013) of Trussell Technology shared logistical factors of implementing WASH systems in vulnerable populations. She shared a specific model of creating a list of all criteria for implementation, bringing the list back to end users for suggested removals and additions, and then considering all criteria, assigning weights, and judging projects using a column system. By converting this system into a radar diagram, the best alternative can be selected. Tiwari explains that this system is necessary to understand individual communities' needs. In developed countries, the work of water and sanitation is not left to individuals, so those implementing solutions may have no idea of the work being placed on primarily women and children. In addition, the cost is heavily subsidized by the government in developed nations, but in the countries where these types of solutions are being implemented, the opposite is true. In fact, it is the vulnerable populations who are responsible for most of the payment as well as the work. Individuals will be expected to implement the solutions, often with no government subsidies. It is thus crucial to use some modeling system to ensure their needs are being met.

Many projects are already underway in these countries. In Addis Ababa, Ethiopia, engineers from the Colorado School of Mines are partnering with Addis Ababa University to account for deteriorating water quantity, increasing sewage efficiency by creating new waste water treatment plants that utilize the wastewater sludge as biogas. By using the wastewater, of which 90% from industry is not treated and 40% is not accounted for after use, engineers are working for a solution to the demand for water (Nigussie, Geza, and Drewes 2013).

In Tanzania, researchers from the Nelson Mandela African Institute of Science and Technology have been constructing wetlands as solutions to sanitation issues. After initial challenges were overcome, the wetlands have been well received. The constructed wetlands provide a strong sense of ownership, fairly straightforward operation and maintenance, and better treatment of wastewater. An operations manual has been created to help with maintenance. Two drawbacks of constructed wetlands are that they provide a good habitat for snakes and they require access to land in order to be built (Njau 2013).

Representatives of OIKOS International discussed a project in Tanzania. They focus on technical and social aspects of making services sustainable. The current four-year project began in March of 2011. The organization has partnered with rural communities, women and school children, and local community organizations. The process to empower entails coordination and full community participation. Some of the challenges have included providing a sense of ownership in the community and some resentment when community members did not realize the work involved (Kajala and Ayo 2013).

In Kenya and Tanzania, for example, PSI, a nongovernmental organization, works to provide safe drinking water for the targeted audience of women, pregnant women, caretakers, and those with AIDS. They train teachers who distribute Waterguard (a point-of-use disinfectant) and instructions for its use. They host behavior-changing community events at shows, clinics, and during household visits to teach proper water-treating techniques, breastfeeding, and handwashing (Mahenge 2013).

The Safe Water and AIDS Project (SWAP) in Kenya is using local community women as long-term change agents. The project works with PSI to distribute Waterguard. SWAP hires women, who are recruited and trained to be entrepreneurs. They are given products to sell in the first round, after which they are in a position to pay to restock inventory for the second and subsequent rounds. The women entrepreneurs visit each household in their catchment once a week to restock Waterguard, and they sell other products. Because they are members of the community, they are more quickly trusted. And, of course, it is also beneficial that they earn money for themselves (Eleveld 2013).

Health

Clean water is basic to health. In cleaning water, chlorine deactivates viruses and bacteria, and protozoa are eliminated with filtration. There are five known ways to clean water: ceramic filtration, chlorination, solar disinfection, biosand filtration, and PuR (water additives.) There is no one-size-fits-all solution—different communities have different needs. Products have been found inappropriate when they are too complicated or have unconvinced users. Solar disinfection, for example, does not work when members of a community believe that hot water is disease ridden. Dr. Daniele Lantagne discussed a successful intervention in Ethiopia, which was attributed to a quality product, distribution, behavior change, and user adoption (Lantagne 2013). Jennifer Foster of PATH (path.org) studies safe water projects to find successful projects. She identifies products to be developed for low-income users, then encourages a system where end users meet with researchers to teach them their needs, and then products are developed and brought back for validation (Foster 2013).

In the research laboratories, the University of Illinois and University of Nairobi are finding ways to clean water. By creating sensors that can detect virus at point of use, the correct water treatment can be used (Madadi et al. 2013). Wastewater treatment plants use chemicals to eliminate pathogens, but they cause many organic by-products or disinfection by-products (DBPs). The chlorine eliminates the DBPs, but of course researchers work to have fewer. Researchers at the University of Illinois and KAUST are working on new strategies to minimize DBPs. In addition, more tests need to be created to find out if more unknown DBPs are being created. Croue and Marinas (2013) explain that we need to find new ways to remove pathogens and minimize toxicity.

In order to create a sustainable ceramic water filtration system, Winston Wole Soboyeja of NM-AIST has created a workshop where local community members make the ceramic filters from local resources. Under the assumption that money must be made to ensure sustainability, the community members locally produce the ceramic filters and sell them to their neighbors (Soboyeja 2013).

Nutrition, Food, and Environment Nexus

In order to meet food security goals, it is crucial to understand the connection between safe water and safe agriculture. There is a limited amount of water, but there are many needs: for drinking, cooking, cleaning, and agriculture. If the food supply is secure, work can be accomplished on water security. In Africa, annual precipitation is fairly good, but water poverty is high because of capacity and governance (Cai 2013). Irrigation is becoming more common there, and it directly affects nutrition, health, and gender. Women are becoming empowered through irrigation, and with empowerment they can sometimes combat poverty. Irrigation, however, causes many negative health consequences, which must be assessed and ameliorated as much as possible before implementation (Ringer 2013).

In West Africa, in Ghana, researchers from the International Water Management Institute are moving from theory to practice by examining how raw sewage is being used for irrigation. Many farmers and nearby families are losing years of life to diarrhea, but the fertilizer does increase crop yields, which supports many jobs, especially for women. By finding a multiple barrier approach for risk reduction from farm to market and through educating consumers, risk is decreased and economic viability is increased, especially for women (Amoah 2013).

Gender Analysis

Table 5.1 provides an overview of select presentations from the summit. We examine three factors that may indicate that gender sensitivity was a part of a project's research design or other aspects of the presenter's work. These factors are (1) consultation with women in the design or implementation of the presented technologies, (2) consideration of the impact of the technology on women, including marginalized women, and (3) whether the interest of people living in locales where the technology is expected to be implemented drives the research agenda.

Out of 25 presentations outlined above, over half (13) do not mention any consultation with women in the design or implementation of their technologies or delivery systems. About half (12) do not mention considering the impact of the technology on women, including marginalized women. While 11 did directly mention impacts on women, few singled out marginalized groups. For an additional two presentations, consideration of the impact of the technology on women was implied. For example, Professor Ximing Cai (2013) from the University of Illinois discussed improving human resources in locales and enhancing the capability of stakeholders by raising awareness. It is implied that women are among these stakeholders.

Finally, we consider whether the interest of people living in locales where technology is expected to be implemented drives presenters' research agenda. This factor is evident in most of the presentations. Only in eight presentations do presenters not directly name the interest of people living in locales and whether they specifically sought out local perspective before designing a project.

SUGGESTIONS FOR FUTURE WORK

Because access to safe household water, improved waste disposal, and sanitation are priorities within communities in East Africa, it is not expected from the outset that attention to gender norms will impede the implementation of the Safe Global Water Network activities. As a part of future research and implementation endeavors, we suggest that researchers and others developing new technologies work with social scientists to meet with male and female stakeholders and hold focus group discussions and interviews with potential users of the new technologies they hope to implement to better learn whether there are gender norms that need to be addressed. In order to prevent potential adverse impacts and/or risks of gender-based exclusion resulting from research and innovation programs, it is important to ask stakeholders and participants in focus group discussions and interviews to consider possible scenarios that could lead to gender-based exclusion, so that producers and implementers of water and sanitation technologies can design and plan to implement programs in a way that would not exacerbate gender inequality.

As noted, the first step to ensure attention to gender equality and female empowerment should be facilitated by directly and systematically consulting with and involving both male and female stakeholders in project design, implementation, and evaluation. To this end, we have identified gender studies units and other relevant female scholars housed in most East African educational institutions (see website: https://docs.google.com/spreadsheets/d/e/2PACX-1vTXeXvNr8yyjsYcdD4n9Rz6T-d-pmK4z0xqC7H4BUDvX6ssjJP5m8IXewSkK1D-pu1v7JKwf4-MgV-h/pubhtml). We propose that engineers invite faculty involved with gender equity issues on these campuses to provide feedback on project design, implementation, and evaluation so as to identify relevant gender gaps and specific ways to reduce them and to serve the needs of both males and females.

It is our recommendation that researchers consort with partner institution faculty who are dedicated to gender equity to conduct a multilevel analysis based on African feminist methodological insights. In addition to academic women's (and men's) participation to conduct the gender analysis, we suggest the solicitation of grassroots involvement.

Another issue to be addressed is how future projects will likely change gender norms and empower women. As for opportunities to enhance grassroots women's participation and leadership, we propose that in future research projects, researchers plan to incorporate women-centered perspectives into project design and implementation via the pre- and post-implementation interviews and focus group discussions. In the pre-implementation data collection phase, it is important to ask women's suggestions for ways to implement the new technologies so that they will be helpful to women in various strata. We will be looking to identify ways to implement the technology so that it will not reproduce gender inequality.

CONCLUSION

The main lessons that an African feminist analysis teaches us about incorporating new safe water and sanitation technologies in African settings are summarized here. In other work, it has been stated (as noted above) that to ensure successful implementation of these technologies for the citizens of East Africa, it is necessary to take "into account sustainability criteria, including social acceptance, technological and physical applicability, economical and institutional aspects, and the need to protect and promote human health and the environment," as in Katukiza et al. (2010, p. 52). Here we have argued that, in addition to these broad criteria, projects should (1) consult with women in the design and/or implementation of the presented technologies, (2) consider the impact of the technology on women, including marginalized women, and (3) ensure that the interest of people living in locales where the technology is expected to be implemented drives the research agenda. Grassroots involvement of women may occur through soliciting their input to project design and seeking their feedback on the effectiveness of new technologies, such as water sensors, treatment processes, and control tools. In chapter 6, we narrow in on the nutrition/food/environment nexus and examine the impact of water and sanitation on early childhood morbidity in Kenya, Tanzania, and Uganda.

NOTE

1. See Appendix 3 for a list of summit participants (speakers).

Chapter Six

Environmental Contamination and Early Childhood Morbidity in Kenya, Tanzania, and Uganda

Assata Zerai, Rebecca L. Morrow, and Courtney Cuthbertson

In this chapter, we explore the effects of water and sanitation quality and availability on early childhood morbidity in East Africa. We present a framework that considers the ways that nation, ethnicity, access to development infrastructure, and other dimensions of oppression intersect to impact the experiences and agency of individuals and groups in accessing safe water and sanitation and reducing early childhood morbidity in Kenya, Tanzania, and Uganda. We analyze recent nationally representative data sets from each country's Demographic and Health Survey (DHS). Drawing from the African feminist framework (Zerai 2014), we argue that safe water, sanitation, and hygiene (WASH) and child health cannot be understood unless socioeconomic, political, and cultural contexts are taken into account. We find not only that safe water and sanitation are in short supply in these countries, but that they also are distributed inequitably and, further, that the lack of these resources has a deleterious effect on early childhood nutrition. It is our hope to contribute to the field of environmental sociology by addressing water and sanitation in an understudied region of the world. Additionally, this work provides results that support child health–related policy recommendations.

ENVIRONMENTAL ENTEROPATHY/ ENVIRONMENTAL ENTERIC DISORDER (EED)[1]

A crucial proximate determinant of chronic malnutrition is environmental contamination. (See Figure 6.1.) In this chapter, we measure environmental contamination using DHS data that indicates household access to improved sanitation (defined by the World Health Organization as flush toilets, ventilated improved pit latrines, pit latrines with slab, and composting toilets, preferably

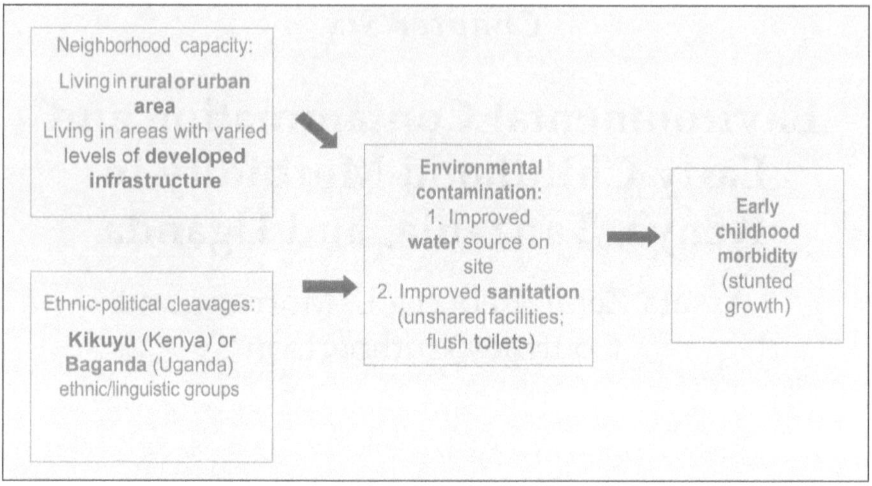

Figure 6.1. Conceptual Model: Factors Affecting Environmental Contamination and Early Childhood Morbidity

all not shared among multiple households, according to DHS 2011), unshared toilet facilities, and improved drinking water available in home or yard. A dominant feature of child health in East Africa is that lack of access to clean drinking water leads to many preventable diseases and even death. Lack of access is affected by a multitude of factors, including breakdown in infrastructure, leading to unreliable piped water sources; drought, leading to inadequate water supply; inadequate sanitation services, leading to contamination of freshwater sources; and floods and climate variability, leading to disastrous water events (Kundzewicz 2013). East Africa is located in a zone subject to unpredictable climate variability (Kundzewicz 2013). Unpredictable climate affects water resources and sanitation, and thus children's health.

The work of Jean Humphrey, Johns Hopkins University researcher and professor of international health, helps us to better understand the import of physical environment to child health. "A key cause of child undernutrition is a disorder of the small intestine known as [environmental] enteropathy, caused by faecal bacteria ingested in large quantities by young children living in conditions of poor sanitation and hygiene" (2009, p. 1032).[2] "Environmental enteropathy is a condition caused by constant contamination and resulting intestinal inflammation. . . . The failure of nutritional interventions and oral vaccines in the developing world may be attributed to [this disorder] . . . due to poor absorption" (Korpe and Petri 2012, p. 328). Humphrey (2009) called for randomized trials to examine environmental enteropathy. Responding to this need, Smith et al. (2013) examined factors related to kwashiorkor, as indicated by stunting among twin pairs in Malawi, and note that "kwashiorkor [is] an enigmatic form of severe acute malnutrition. [It] is the consequence of inadequate nutrient intake plus additional environmental insults" (p. 548). Smith and her colleagues found that environmental enteropathy predicts impaired growth and development, also known as stunting, among children.

Undernourished children have an abnormal gut microbiome; according to Smith and colleagues, "[t]he combination of Malawian diet and kwashiorkor microbiome produced marked weight loss" (2013, p. 548). The abnormal microbiomes, researchers found, stay the same even if better food is provided. In twin pairs, half of the children had abnormal microbiomes and half had normal ones; even with the same food supplementation, the children with the deleterious bacteria in their intestines were not able to gain appropriate weight for their age. Poor sanitation and hygiene plus fecal contamination in the domestic environment altered the intestinal bacteria.

Environmental contamination leads to environmental enteropathy that creates malnutrition through malabsorption regardless of increased quality of nutritional supplementation. Mbuya and Humphrey introduce the idea of "baby-WASH interventions (sanitation and water improvement, handwashing with soap, ensuring a clean play and infant feeding environment and food hygiene) that interrupt specific pathways through which feco-oral transmission occurs in the first two years of a child's life" (2016, p. 106). Further, WASH interventions must be targeted to appropriately reduce EED.

Given that environmental enteric dysfunction (EED) is estimated to affect a third of children in developing countries (Mbuya and Humphrey 2016), stopping infants' and children's ingestion of EED pathogens using WASH interventions may help significantly reduce stunting around the world (Mbuya and Humphrey 2016). There is overwhelming evidence of the importance of handwashing in water-scarce areas.[3] In a 2007–2009 study of 185 Kenyan schools, investigators found that WASH interventions in water-scarce schools decreased odds of diarrhea compared to control schools (Dreibelbis et al. 2014).

Some recent criticisms of WASH interventions have been levied[4] by those promoting the "hygiene hypothesis." We briefly address those here. According to Bloomfield et al. (2006), "[t]he 'hygiene hypothesis' as originally formulated by Strachan proposes that a cause of the recent rapid rise in atopic disorders could be a lower incidence of infection in early childhood, transmitted by unhygienic contact with older siblings. Use of the term 'hygiene hypothesis' has led to several interpretations, some of which are not supported by a broader survey of the evidence" (p. 402). So the "hygiene hypothesis" or the "microbial exposure hypothesis" addresses impacts on atopic diseases (Bloomfield et al. 2006; Ring, Krämer, and Behrendt 2004) and respiratory infections (Ring, Krämer, and Behrendt 2004). It does not challenge the fact that the subclinical condition of environmental enteropathy is associated with hygienic conditions in farming areas and, in particular, with exposure of young children to animal waste. Nor does it challenge associations between environmental contamination and growth stunting.[5]

Researchers have signaled the importance of sanitation beyond diarrheal intervention by pointing to the impact of environmental contamination on abnormal gut biomes. Higher rates of exposure to livestock, especially poultry, may be related to stunting in children as they increase risks for environmental enteric disorder (EED), diarrhea, and respiratory infections (Headey and Hirvonen 2016).

Headey and Hirvonen (2016) measure the relative impact of a positive benefit to children's growth that accrues from families owning poultry and livestock with the potentially negative effect of keeping poultry and other livestock in the home overnight. In rural Ethiopia, poultry ownership has been positively associated with children's height-for-age; however, if poultry is kept indoors overnight, there is a negative association with children's height-for-age (significant only for poultry and not for other animals). This is likely due to increased infection risk.

The positive effects of poultry ownership interpreted in conjunction with the negative effects of close physical exposure to poultry point to the need for attention to hygiene as an area for intervention in the relationship between owning poultry and healthy child development (Headey and Hirvonen 2016).

> Although these associations should not be interpreted too literally, the negative association between close physical exposure to poultry and child growth is large in magnitude, and not statistically different in magnitude from the positive association between poultry ownership and growth. This result suggests that poultry-related hygiene issues are an important mediating factor linking poultry ownership to child growth. (p. 11)

WASH interventions are enabled to have broader impacts when considered through the lens of both health and development (Loevinsohn et al. 2015). For example, Loevinsohn et al. (2015) argue that efforts to ensure food security must also address micronutrient deficiencies to create health by lessening vulnerability to illness and infection. Previous work has also found that mothers' education is related to their children's nutritional status and health (Smith et al. 2013). Through education, women are able to "make better use of water and sanitation infrastructure, thereby gaining health benefits for their children (Jalan and Ravallion 2003)" (as cited in Loevinsohn et al. 2015, p. 660). Water governance, including avoidance of contamination that puts health at risk, can be effective at the local level (Loevinsohn et al. 2015).

Supported by this evidence, the African feminist framework utilized in this book recognizes contextual factors (as argued in Zerai 2014). At the household level, *children's* behavior (including crawling and possibly picking up contaminants) and *families'* work to provide for and protect their children are mediated by their access to *social institutions* (such as schools,[6] churches, and health care facilities), by the *state* (at local, regional, and national levels—often directly responsible for infrastructure to deliver safe water and sanitation), and by *global/multinational entities* (UN, WHO, IMF/World Bank, and multinational commercial interests), all of which may contribute to disease vectors related to environmental contamination. "Ensuring universal access to potable water and plumbing would render the sequelae of environmental enteropathy obsolete" (Korpe and Petri 2012, p. 334).

However, in this chapter, we examine effects of environmental contamination on early childhood morbidity.[7] This allows us to shed light on structural impediments to child health.

WATER AND SANITATION

Water and sanitation are important factors affecting morbidity, and growth-stunting in particular, that operate through environmental contamination. Here we analyze the DHS data sets from Kenya, Tanzania, and Uganda for the following years: Kenya, 2008–2009; Tanzania, 2010; Uganda 2011. These data show that children in all three settings have low heights for their age, reflecting chronic malnutrition (32% in Uganda, 35% in Kenya, 42% in Tanzania).

Figure 6.1 depicts a conceptual model that features environmental contamination as an important proximate determinant of chronic malnutrition. Our analysis shows that a lack of access to clean drinking water and proper sanitation leads to child morbidity, as measured by chronic malnutrition resulting in stunted growth (low height for age). Inequality is captured in the model by the inclusion of neighborhood capacity and ethnicity.[8]

Before discussing our results, we first examine factors related to water and sanitation availability. Then, we test a partial model to examine effects of access to improved proximate sources of drinking water and flush toilets in residence (as a proxy for environmental contamination) on early childhood morbidity (as measured by low height-for-age among children ages 3 to 59 months) in Kenya, Tanzania, and Uganda.

Table 6.1 provides details concerning the availability of drinking water on the premises of households in Kenya, Tanzania, and Uganda from description of data to be analyzed here and from DHS country reports. Improved sources of drinking water may be available in the home or in the yard. As you can see, examining water available in residence shows water resources to be scarce in the vast majority of children's households. Only 30% of households in Kenya and 26% in Tanzania have access to improved sources of drinking

Table 6.1. Drinking Water Availability in Kenya, Tanzania, and Uganda

	Kenya 2014	*Tanzania 2015–2016*	*Uganda 2011*
Drinking water on premises: all households	29.8% (71.3%)	25.6%	6.4%
In urban areas	59.4% (88.2%)	41.0%	27.9%
In improved infrastructure areas	Nairobi 60.3%	Kilimanjaro 40.4% Zanzibar 33.3%	Kampala 35.6%
By ethnicity	Kikuyu 62.9%	N/A**	Baganda 11.1%
No. of households	19,564	9,736	9,033

Sources: Country Reports (data in parentheses) from 2014 DHS for Kenya; 2010 DHS for Tanzania; and 2011 DHS for Uganda; as well as analysis of the 2014 DHS for Kenya, 2015–2016 DHS for Tanzania, and 2011 DHS for Uganda.

*Drinking water may be available on premises in these forms: piped into dwelling, piped into yard/plot, or protected well/spring in yard/plot (Measure DHS 2011, 2014, 2016).

**Ethnicity data is not available in the TDHS.

water on their premises, and in Uganda, fewer than 10% of households have in-residence access. As is expected, there is greater access to drinking water on the premises of households in urban areas. Twice as many households in Kenya have this access, and in Uganda, more than four times as many urban households have access to drinking water on their premises.

Areas with improved infrastructure—such as Nairobi proper in Kenya, Kilimanjaro and Zanzibar in Tanzania, and Kampala in Uganda—have even greater access to safe water on site. In Nairobi, twice as many residents have access to water in residence as do the DHS households in the entire country. Significant ethnic differences exist in Kenya (Ndiritu et al. 2016) and Uganda (Green 2010a, 2010b).[9] Of Kikuyu in Kenya, 63% of households had access to water on site, which is more than twice as many households in the Kenya data set. And in Uganda, touted by some as "the most ethnically fractionalized country in the world" (Green 2010a, 11), 60% of children's households in the Baganda ethnic group were in the two wealthiest quartiles, and the Baganda group had a larger percentage of households with access to improved water sources relative to the country as a whole.[10] Water resources clearly are not distributed equitably throughout these countries.

Flush toilets are also scarce. "Prevention of [environmental] enteropathy will be crucial to normalize child growth, and this will not be possible without provision of toilets" (Humphrey 2009, p. 1034). Table 6.2 shows the percentages of households in each country overall that has access to flush toilets, improved sanitation, as well as those that do not have toilet facilities.[11] In Kenya's 2014 DHS, more urban households have flush toilets relative to the rest of the country. In Tanzania, a greater share of urban residents has access to flush toilets than do counterparts in the rest of the country. And in Uganda, more than four times as many urban residents have flush toilets in their households. So, unfor-

Table 6.2. Sanitation Facilities in Kenya, Tanzania, and Uganda

	Kenya 2014	*Tanzania 2015–2016*	*Uganda 2011*
In-country flush toilets*	6.6%	12.9%	1.8%
Improved sanitation*	24.0%	27.6%	16.4%
With no facilities	15.4%	13.1%	9.7%
Urban flush toilets	25.7%	39.9%	8.6%
Flush toilets in improved-infrastructure areas	Nairobi 33.9%	Zanzibar 17.9% Kilimanjaro 23.0%	Kampala 16.4%
Flush toilets by ethnicity	Kikuyu 24.5%	Data unavailable	Baganda 11.1%
No. of households	16,549	9,590	9,033

Sources: Country Reports from 2014 DHS for Kenya; 2016 DHS for Tanzania; and 2011 DHS for Uganda; as well as analysis of 2014 DHS for Kenya, 2015–2016 DHS for Tanzania, and 2011 DHS for Uganda.
*Flush toilets and improved sanitation are the percentages of households with unshared facilities.

tunately, as with water resources, the distribution of flush toilets to households is not equitable within these countries. For Kenya and Tanzania, these inequalities are even more severe when considering residence in areas with improved infrastructure. Ethnicity is an important cleavage in Kenya and Uganda, as Kikuyu households and Baganda households are more likely to have flush toilets. We can now take a step beyond this descriptive overview of inequitable access and examine whether these differences are statistically significant.

WATER AVAILABILITY AND UNSHARED FLUSHED TOILETS IN RESIDENCE

Kenya

Table 6.3 provides logistic regression results for drinking water available in residence[12] and for flush toilets in Kenya. The first section depicts results from logistic regression analyses of water piped or other improved sources in residence that provides further evidence of the inequitable distribution of this resource. In Kenya, access to water is increased by living in urban areas, belonging to the Kikuyu ethnicity, and living in Nairobi. Children from ages 3 to 59 months living in urban areas are more than three times as likely as children living in rural areas to have water available in their residence. Kikuyu children are 4.6 times as likely to have drinking water on site. And children living in Nairobi are 1.7 times as likely to have water piped or other improved sources in their home or yard. All variables are significant at the $\alpha = .001$ level. Analyses of flushed toilets include the same covariates: urban residence, Kikuyu ethnic group membership, and Nairobi residence. These three variables have a positive association with flush toilets in residence. Results for both dependent variables

Table 6.3. Kenya: Logistic Regressions for Water and Sanitation, 2011

Water at home	*Exp (B)*	
Urban	3.186	***
Kikuyu	4.590	***
Nairobi	1.664	***
Constant	.183	***
Improved sanitation	*Exp (B)*	
Urban	21.665	***
Kikuyu	1.598	***
Nairobi	1.427	***
Constant	.007	***

Source: Analysis of 2014 DHS for Kenya.
Note: According to the World Health Organization/UNICEF Joint Monitoring Programme for Water Supply and Sanitation, improved sanitation includes flush toilets, ventilated improved pit latrines, pit latrines with slab, and composting/Ecosan toilets, preferably all not shared (Uganda Bureau of Statistics [UBOS] and Institute for Resource Development/Macro Systems 2011).

show a clear preference for Kikuyu ethnicity, even when controlling for both urban and Nairobi residence.

Tanzania

Table 6.4 provides similar results in the country of Tanzania, in which living in Zanzibar, Kilimanjaro, or urban areas increases access to drinking water in residence. All variables are significant at the $\alpha = .001$ level. Logistic regression analysis of drinking water available at home and flushed toilets include urban residence and notable regions (Kilimanjaro and Zanzibar, with the rest of the mainland as omitted category) as covariates. There is a clear preference for urban areas and Kilimanjaro or Zanzibar residence for both resources. All variables are positively associated with flush toilets on premises.

Uganda

Finally, in the first section of Table 6.5, logistic regression results show that living in urban areas and belonging to Baganda ethnicity are associated with water accessibility in Uganda. Both variables are significant at the $\alpha = .001$ level. All three variables, including Kampala residence, have a positive association with improved sanitation. Living in Kampala increases by 1.8 times the likelihood that children's households have improved sanitation. Young

Table 6.4. Tanzania: Logistic Regressions for Water and Sanitation, 2015–2016

Water at home	*Exp (B)*	
Zanzibar	1.810	*
Kilimanjaro	1.720	**
Urban	2.656	***
Constant	.258	***
Improved sanitation	*Exp (B)*	
Zanzibar	24.556	***
Kilimanjaro	5.296	***
Urban	23.130	***
Constant	.111	***

Source: Analysis of 2015–16 DHS for Tanzania.
Note: According to the World Health Organization/UNICEF Joint Monitoring Programme for Water Supply and Sanitation, improved sanitation includes flush toilets, ventilated improved pit latrines, pit latrines with slab, and composting/Ecosan toilets, preferably all not shared (Uganda Bureau of Statistics [UBOS] and Institute for Resource Development/Macro Systems 2011).

Table 6.5. Uganda: Logistic Regressions for Water and Sanitation, 2011

Water at home	*Exp (B)*	
Kampala	1.146	N.S.
Baganda	1.586	***
Urban	8.098	***
Constant	.047	***
Improved sanitation	*Exp (B)*	
Kampala	1.826	***
Baganda	3.408	***
Urban	4.777	***
Constant	.210	***

Source: Analysis of 2011 DHS for Uganda.
Note: According to the World Health Organization/UNICEF Joint Monitoring Programme for Water Supply and Sanitation, improved sanitation includes flush toilets, ventilated improved pit latrines, pit latrines with slab, and composting/Ecosan toilets, preferably all not shared (Uganda Bureau of Statistics [UBOS] and Institute for Resource Development/Macro Systems 2011).

children with Baganda ethnicity are 3.4 times as likely to have improved sanitation in their homes, and living in urban areas more than quadruples the likelihood of improved sanitation in the household. All three variables are significant at the $\alpha = .001$ level. Notably, Baganda ethnicity is significant in all models, even when controlling for urban and Kampala residence.

WATER, SANITATION, AND CHILD HEALTH

While water resources and sanitation were clearly distributed, with preference given to urban areas, the next question to ask is whether water and sanitation resources affect children's nutritional intake. We analyze determinants of chronic malnutrition among infants and children (ages 3–59 months) in East Africa. Table 6.6 shows results of children's anthropometric measurements of weight-for-age, weight-for-height, and height-for-age in data available from the Demographic and Health Surveys. The number of children experiencing stunting (indicating chronic malnutrition) in Kenya has decreased from 36% in 2003 to 26% in 2014. In Tanzania, there has been a decrease in stunting, from 44% in 2004–2005 to 34% in 2015–2016, and in Uganda there has been a decrease from nearly 45% in 2000–2001 to 33% in 2011.

Logistic regression results in Table 6.7 analyze growth faltering (specifically, stunted growth), measured as a dichotomous dependent variable looking at the extent to which individual-level determinants and community

Table 6.6. Nutrition Status in East Africa: Percentages of Children Ages 3 to 59 Months with Low Height-for-Age, Weight-for-Height, and Weight-for-Age

	Data Source	*Height-for-Age (Below −2 SD; Total % Stunted)*	*Weight-for-Height (Below −2 SD; Total % Wasting [Too Thin])*	*Weight-for-Age (Below −2 SD; Total % Growth-Faltering)*
Kenya	2014 DHS	26.0	4.0	11.0
	2008–09 DHS	35.3	6.7	16.1
	2003 DHS	35.7	6.0	15.8
Tanzania	2015–16 DHS	34.4	4.4	13.5
	2010 DHS	42.0	4.8	15.8
	2004–05 DHS	44.3	3.5	16.4
Uganda	2011 DHS	33.4	4.7	13.8
	2006 DHS	38.1	6.1	15.9
	2000–01 DHS	44.8	4.9	18.4

Sources: ICF International 2012.

*Percentages of children under 5 years classified as malnourished according to WHO standards of three anthropometric indexes of nutritional status: height-for-age, weight-for-height, and weight-for-age, by country and all survey years for which data is collected.

Table 6.7. Logistic Regressions for Effect of Water and Sanitation on Stunting among Children Ages 3 to 59 Months in Kenya (2014), Tanzania (2015–2016), and Uganda (2011)

Kenya			*Tanzania*			*Uganda*		
Stunting	*Exp (B)*		*Stunting*	*Exp (B)*		*Stunting*	*Exp (B)*	
Urban	.768	***	Urban	.586	***	Urban	.657	*
Kikuyu	.875	*	Zanzibar	.543	N.S.	Baganda	1.065	N.S.
Nairobi	.993	N.S.	Kilimanjaro	.781	N.S.	Kampala	.471	*
Improved sanitation	.810	***	Improved sanitation	1.510	***	Improved sanitation	.838	N.S.
Toilet facilities not shared with other households	.964	*	Toilet facilities shared with other households	1.024	N.S.	Toilet facilities shared with other households	.912	N.S.
Water piped into residence	.706	***	Water piped into residence	.977	N.S.	Water piped into residence	.724	N.S.
Constant	.439	***	Constant	.347	***	Constant	.585	***

Source: Analysis of 2014 DHS for Kenya, 2015–2016 DHS for Tanzania, and 2011 DHS for Uganda.

conditions affect the growth of young children ages 3 to 59 months (all children measured in KDHS, TDHS, and UDHS). For each country, a child's lack of access to sanitation is related to stunting. We posit that unsafe water and sanitation work through mechanisms such as environmental enteropathy, which impact the expected gains from nutrition.

WATER, SANITATION, AND CHILD MORBIDITY

Consistent with the findings of Smith et al. (2013), access to clean water and improved sanitation, serving as a proxy for reduced environmental contamination, is associated with a lower prevalence of chronic malnutrition, as evidenced by stunting among children 3 to 59 months of age in Kenya and Tanzania. In Kenya, improved sanitation decreased the odds of stunting by .810 ($\alpha < .001$), and unshared facilities decreased odds by .964 ($\alpha < .05$). In Tanzania, children without flush toilets were 1.69 times as likely to experience chronic malnutrition as those with flush toilets ($\alpha = .001$). Water available in residence decreased the odds of low height-for-age by .715 in Kenya ($\alpha < .001$) and by .721 in Tanzania ($\alpha < .05$).

Uganda has focused on improved sanitation to ensure that more households would benefit (versus spending funds for fewer groups to obtain flush toilets), so we examined improved sanitation and not just flush toilets in the Uganda child health model. The results are that in Uganda, the odds of growth faltering within households that had access to improved water and sanitation facilities and those with families of Baganda ethnicity *were not statistically significant*. This exciting result shows that Uganda's efforts to achieve the Millennium Development Goal of improved access to sanitation are paying off with lowered child morbidity for all. For all three countries, living in urban areas decreased the odds of stunting under the age of 5. And living in Kampala, of the 3 more developed areas considered, decreased odds of stunting among children under the age of 5.

The realities of the overall low levels of water and sanitation require redress to improve the health of children in Kenya, Tanzania, and Uganda, with equitable access to clean water and sanitation as important components. Certainly, adequate nutrition and access to health services are also required. Recent literature shows evidence that a direct association between hygienic conditions (as proxied by access to improved water and sanitation) and growth faltering is likely to be complicated by other factors, such as mother's education, household socioeconomic status, infrastructure, nutritional intake, and others (as shown in Headey and Hirvonen 2016).[13] In future work we will examine these additional factors, and we will conduct qualitative studies in-country to gain a better understanding of household contaminants and ways to effectively implement baby-WASH interventions.

Our results point to the necessity of conceptualizing early childhood morbidity within a holistic environmental context, including not only the child and her or his immediate physical surroundings but also household and community factors. National interventions that promote equity in access have far-reaching effects, as shown by results from Uganda. While international/global interventions have the potential to exert a positive impact, as has been shown by Millenium Development Goals, Sustainable Development Goals, and the Reproductive Maternal, Newborn and Child Health Program, an integrated approach is needed (Griffiths 2013; Humphrey 2009; Korpe and Petri 2012; Kundzewicz 2013, Smith et al. 2013) to continue to improve the water, sanitation, and health of children in Kenya, Tanzania, and Uganda. Clean water is enabled through adequate quality and quantity, and sanitation is enabled through appropriate technologies. In future work, it would be useful to examine the impact of health education, including new baby-WASH interventions.

NOTES

1. An earlier version of this section on environmental enteropathy was published by Zerai (2014). For a fuller explanation of environmental enteropathy/environmental enteric disorder (EED), see Mbuya and Humphrey 2016.

2. Environmental enteropathy is also known as environmental enteric disorder, or EED (Watanabe and Petri 2016).

3. Of course, evidence of the importance of handwashing to prevent the spread of influenza also abounds (e.g., Meilicke et al. 2008).

4. For examples see White 2014 and Bloomfield et al. 2006.

5. For recent studies pointing to this association, see Prendergast and Humphrey 2015 and Mbuya and Humphrey 2016.

6. One study shows that even the tap flow quality and physical cleanliness of wash facilities are associated with improved handwashing behavior in educational settings (Mariwah, Hampshire, and Wasim 2012).

7. Another disease vector to consider is malaria. We chose not to include this in our analyses, however, for several reasons. First, lack of sufficient nutritional intake and not malaria is found to be the predominant cause of growth faltering (Matanda, Mittelmark, and Kigaru 2014). According to Friedman et al. (2005), the complicated relationship between undernutrition and malaria-related morbidity (also corroborated by Caulfield, Richard, and Black 2004) in Kenya follows: "[T]he relationship between malaria and protein-energy malnutrition is controversial" (p. 698, as are all quotes in this endnote). To examine "whether undernutrition is associated with increased or decreased malaria attributable morbidity," researchers collected data "on nutritional status, recent history of clinical illness, socioeconomic status, current

malaria infection status, and hemoglobin." Though "the cross-sectional nature of the study limits the interpretation of causality," researchers' "data provide[d] . . . observational support that the presence of undernutrition, in particular chronic undernutrition, places children at higher, not lower risk of malaria-related morbidity." Second, we ran analysis to examine malaria in an earlier iteration and found that effects of water and sanitation were not statistically significant.

8. Though maternal characteristics such as mother's education, literacy, and health literacy are shown to be significant in the literature, health literacy would be most salient (Makoka and Masibo 2015) regarding the association of environmental contamination and stunting. Unfortunately, this variable is not captured in the Demographic and Health Studies.

9. "Nyerere's commitment to his ideal state forcefully downplayed the role of ethnic association in public life and instead accentuated a Tanzanian national identity" (Malipula 2014, 61). While ethnicity is a central cleavage on much of the African continent, "Tanzanian society is not structured by this cleavage" (Malipula 2014, p. 49).

10. While much work needs to be done to unpack dimensions of power and ethnicity in Uganda, a signal to this relationship can be found in the historical use of the patronage system to maintain political power. For example, "In order to placate . . . the Baganda, Museveni has thus kept a regular amount of patronage flowing to them via posts in the armed forces, the cabinet (which includes an ever-increasing number of 'presidential advisors'), and various semi-autonomous government agencies (Mwenda and Tangri 2005; Tangri and Mwenda 2001) as cited in Green (2010b). For details on sources within the quote, see the original text.

11. To define improved toilets: "A household is classified as having an improved toilet if the toilet is used only by household members and if the toilet separates the waste from human contact (WHO and UNICEF, 2010). Flush/pour toilets that flush to a piped sewer system, and ventilated improved pit (VIP) latrines, pit latrines with a slab, and composting toilets (which separate solid waste from water) are also classified as improved toilets" (Uganda Bureau of Statistics and Institute for Resource Development/Macro Systems 2011, p. 13). In the Uganda data set, flush and pour toilets are captured in one variable, so improved toilets and not flush toilets are used in Uganda models. (For details on sources within the quote, see the original text.)

12. Drinking water may be available on premises in the following forms: piped into dwelling, piped into yard/plot, or protected well/spring in yard/plot (Uganda Bureau of Statistics [UBOS] and Institute for Resource Development/Macro Systems 2011; National Bureau of Statistics (NBS) [Tanzania] and ICF Macro 2011; Kenya National Bureau of Statistics, Ministry of Health/Kenya, National AIDS Control Council/Kenya, Kenya Medical Research Institute, National Council for Population and Development/Kenya, and ICF International 2015; Ministry of Health, Community Development, Gender, Elderly and Children—MoHCDGEC/Tanzania Mainland, Ministry of Health—MoH/Zanzibar, National Bureau of Statistics—NBS/Tanzania, Office of Chief Government Statistician—OCGS/Zanzibar, and ICF 2016).

13. According to Headey and Hirvonen (2016), it is important to consider whether the household owns poultry and the location of poultry (whether they are kept in house at night). Other relevant factors may be whether household members own other livestock and whether livestock are kept in house. In their work, the authors consider control factors such as education, household assets, land size, and iron roof, in addition to household characteristics that we examine as environmental contamination factors, such as use of improved toilets and safe water. They also examine access to electricity, floor material type, nutrition knowledge, health worker visits, and agricultural worker visits.

Conclusion

Paying Serious Attention to Women's Scholarship to Influence Policy in East Africa

Assata Zerai and Joanna B. Perez

A crucial source of social change in Kenya, Tanzania, and Uganda has been the efforts of mothers, health professionals, and activists to advocate for clean water, safe sanitation, and the health of its citizenry. In all these efforts, those seeking lasting, sustainable, and socially conscious change have focused on comprehensive transformations based on addressing structural inequality. In this chapter, we pay serious attention to women's scholarship that may influence water and sanitation technology and policy in East Africa. We end by reviewing the demands for safe water and sanitation from women in East African communities and providing a recap of lessons from an African feminist analysis of water and sanitation in East Africa that inform family-centered policy.

AFRICAN FEMINISM

African feminism (Gaidzanwa 1997; Mama 2002; Zerai 2014) articulates women-centered perspectives that describe intersecting oppressions and privileges of African women's and girls' lived experiences as well as the social structures in which they are situated. Zerai (2014) and Zerai, Perez, and Wang (2016) developed an African feminist *methodology* built on women's scholarship and activism. Here we challenge a structural factor operating as a mechanism that impedes the development of African feminist thought and decelerate its uptake by delineating female scholars in East African universities who should be consulted in subsequent work. It is our opinion that encumbered access to improved water and sanitation technology among women in especially impoverished rural and unplanned urban settlement areas in East Africa creates barriers to women's empowerment and their involvement in national discourse and strategic planning for development. To address this problem, it is important to be intentional about seeking female scholars' perspectives on the design and implementation of development infrastructure.

Given the centrality of African women's role in society, economic growth, domestic labor, and primary care, we argue that leaving African women out of the conversation may be partly responsible for the pervasiveness of neoliberalism today. Zerai and Banks (2002) have argued that pursuing African feminism provides the opportunity to create intellectual tools to build toward social justice instead of reproducing master narratives. Without the intellectual diversity that African feminism offers, capital expansion and subsequent development, even in the wake of social movements and protest, morph not into something liberatory but something predatory. For example, in terms of building an infrastructure for development, "public management" is an approach to government and nonprofit administration that resembles private-sector management. In particular, it emphasizes tools that maximize efficiency and effectiveness. However, public management approaches are controversial because "efficiency" is prioritized over meeting the needs of the most marginalized members of society.

> From the end of the 1970s to the 1990s, . . . governments around the world were engaged in widespread and sustained reforms of their public administration. These reforms were born out of economic recession, but also had political and social drivers. They were initiated by the political apex and fuelled by New Right ideology. Collectively, these reforms came to be termed New Public Management (NPM). . . . NPM is characterised by marketisation, privatisation, managerialism, performance measurement and accountability. This employment of corporate attitudes in public administration is grounded on certain theories, mainly public choice, transaction cost analysis and principal–agent theory. (Tolofari 2005)

In some well-endowed contexts of East Africa, improved access to water and sanitation promises to contribute to enhanced quality of life (Tsinda, Abbott, and Chenoweth 2015). But in these spaces, we continue to see disparate access, especially along the lines of socioeconomic status, educational background, language, and family structure (Amuyunzu-Nyamongo and Ezeh 2005). Consequently, residents of East African communities suffering from informal housing, population density, and lack of water and sanitation facilities are more susceptible to suffer from various illnesses (Penrose et al. 2010; Blanton et al. 2015; Breiman et al. 2015). The social conditions experienced by these residents and future generations threaten their development, health, and mortality rates (Machiwa 2003; Beguy, Mumah, and Gottschalk 2014; Olack et al. 2014). Given the crucial need to revitalize these communities, some drivers of innovation aim to provide water and sanitation as public goods, while others seek to capitalize on what they see as their intellectual property. In emerging markets, where centralized development infrastructure to provide water access and sanitation is challenging, new technology is surging ahead, and principles of neoliberal market-driven expansion may trump any efforts to reign in, centrally manage, tax, and ensure nondiscrimination in access to what potentially could be a public good (as shown in chapter 3). At the same time, through policy reform and community organizing, residents of East African communities are mobilizing to change their social conditions and position (Magigi and Majani 2006; Hooper 2012).

African feminist principles present an alternative perspective in line with a bottom-up approach that is informed by the values of social justice, equity, diversity, and inclusion and that eschews heteronormativity, ableism, religious chauvinism, exclusive nationalisms, and marginalization of underrepresented groups from access to technology. Access to water and sanitation technology is a major public management issue of the 21st century. Without it, members of emerging economies will continue to suffer ill effects.

How can attention to the experiences of African women and postcolonial feminist scholarship provide a unique perspective on enhancing access to improved water and sanitation? Herein, we emphasize the voices of women and show how their framings are important when we examine science and technology in society. Women's lack of access to new water and sanitation technology and planning for its distribution without considering women or consulting with them leads to fundamental design flaws and slow uptake among women. Inaccessible new water and sanitation technologies may result in dire consequences for women in East African settings and their families.

THE COST OF EXCLUDING AFRICAN WOMEN

The problem that this chapter addresses is that Western researchers often do not incorporate the voices of African women in their research endeavors, and a serious engagement in women's empowerment and improving access to water and sanitation for women and their families cannot happen without this preliminary step. Building from Frantz Fanon (1968) and Lewis Gordon (2006), Reiland Rabaka (2010) refers to this as *epistemic apartheid*, "a process of critical decay within a field or discipline" (Gordon 2006) due to its lack of intellectual diversity. Rabaka further describes this process as one "of institutional racism [and] academic colonization and conceptual quarantining of knowledge, anti-imperial thought, and/or radical political praxis produced and presented by . . . 'especially black' intellectual-activists" (2010, p. 16). To Rabaka's description, we add "especially" African (and other non-Western) *women* intellectual-activists. We ask, How do we engage the scholarship and activism of African women to ensure that their voices and perspectives inform research on development, especially when this research is focused on African contexts? We utilize an African feminist approach to promote intellectual diversity encompassing perspectives from Africa and the African diaspora.

The words, theoretical perspectives, research, and political activity of women in African contexts have been obscured from Western researchers. Their important potential contributions remain inaccessible due to the difficulties and resources needed in order to publish their work in Western and top-tier international journals. It is our task to break down these barriers and bring to the fore the efforts of African women—both academic and activist—to provide health and healing.

METHODOLOGY

The UNESCO and International Social Science Council World Report in 2010 articulated 21st-century priorities and expounded the need to address knowledge divides between scholars in the Southern hemisphere and North Atlantic researchers. They explain that Africa is affected by the structural and epistemic disparities that produce the knowledge divides (Harrison 2016). These divides separate and marginalize the Global South, especially women in those settings, and intersectional perspectives help us to understand that they can take place and multiplicatively affect people living in rural areas; in underdeveloped provinces in countries on the African continent (Zerai 2014; Henderson, Zerai, and Morrow, 2017); and between core and periphery communities within a town such as Mombasa suburbs versus Mombasa slums or refugee settlements. We present a methodology to break down those divides, as discussed in Chapter 5. Following the example of Zerai (2014), we examined the available online curricula vitae of all female university scholars in Kenya, Tanzania and Uganda, and we created a database with links to their publications and papers (https://docs.google.com/spreadsheets/d/e/2PACX-1vTXeXvNr8yyjsYcdD4n9Rz6T-dpmK4z0xqC7H4BUDvX6ssjJP5m8IXewSkK1D-pu1v7JKwf4-MgV-h/pubhtml). This multistep process has begun with English language publications. To broaden our scope, in subsequent work we will examine publications in other languages, websites, and other reports. It is our hope to join to inspire the building of a database of postcolonial women scholars throughout the world in the long term.

SUMMARY AND LESSONS FROM FEMALE SCHOLARS IN EAST AFRICA

We must seek to disrupt the conventional division of labor, in which African communities provide only the raw resources to make technology (West 2016) and the markets to buy it (the focus of the emerging water and technology industry). Answering UNESCO's call (UNESCO and International Social Science Council 2010) to work in dialogue with intellectuals and practitioners in the southern hemisphere is a crucial intervention if we want to stem the process of critical decay within technological innovation that is resulting from their lack of intellectual diversity. For many of us, humanity's big questions inspire our academic pursuits. Moving beyond our limited understandings requires including marginalized groups. Solving the problem of inadequate water and sanitation globally requires a free flow of ideas that eschews marginalization of women in the global south. This cannot happen if we continue to reify transnational and gendered digital divides. A reimagining of water and technology design, production, and distribution that places women at the center may help us build a stable bridge to close the gap and resolve the issue.

While we have included scholarship of women from East Africa (as authors and in citations) throughout this work, we thought it fitting to assess our conclusions from the perspectives offered by women in our database. We summarize conclusions from our publication that are consistent with the work of female scholars located in East African universities. In future work, we will excavate the writings of women who are not easily located in common Western databases to examine ways in which they support or challenge these conclusions. We end by identifying new areas of inquiry prompted by book chapters and by female East African scholars.

- A social justice advocacy framework is an appropriate orientation to increase fairness in the distribution of crucial resources, such as improved water and sanitation, to target communities in East Africa.
- In order to improve educational outcomes for girls, improved water and sanitation are necessary both in households and in schools.
- Access or lack of access to water and sanitation permeates every aspect of women's and girls' lives in East Africa. A feminist intervention into the critical development studies framework is needed to ensure that gender equity is taken into account in development strategies and to ensure that a rubric of development effectiveness is intentionality to avoid reproducing inequality.
- Multinational corporation actors' and local elites' roles in development must be examined critically. Vigilant critical inquiry to consider roles of all actors, as well as development strategies that stamp out exploitation by multinational interests and corruption on the part of elites, is crucial to the success of development plans.
- Historical and contemporary factors have led to the maldistribution of safe water and sanitation infrastructure in East Africa, including the uneven development instigated as part of the region's colonial heritage, the influences of multinational corporations, economic structural adjustment

programs, the tourism industry, failing development infrastructure, and incursions by nongovernmental organizations.

- Given that several aspects of the education provided at public schools render it a sexist, repressive tool that limits women's ability to critically examine the social conditions and hierarchies created by contemporary, historical, indigenous, and colonial political and religious authorities, critical educational tools emanating from existing indigenous and customary systems of learning can provide solutions that are relevant to improving the lives of women, and they must be integrated into public schools.
- Concerning water basin management, land rent and water user fees should be merged to ease the process of revenue collection and promote cost-effective allocation of water rights. Linkages between the ownership of the landholders/schemes and the water rights system will strengthen the decentralization system from central to local government and law enforcement by the Pangani Basin Water Office. This will enhance the revenue collection system and joint planning and budgeting between PBWO and local government authorities.
- Providing adequate safe water, sanitation, and hygiene (WASH) services and facilities requires political will and commitment of country resources to increase budgets for water supply and infrastructure. Priority of the domestic water supply should be clearly stipulated in the water rights system.
- Women must be engaged fully in planning and decision making to ensure that families have access to adequate WASH services and facilities. WASH investment should also be implemented as a package that reflects other basic necessities (such as education, energy, and shelter) to promote welfare of women and children.
- In projects to design and implement new water and sanitation technologies, researchers, corporate actors, and others should (1) consult with women in target settings in the design and/or implementation of the presented technologies, (2) consider the impact of the technology on women, including marginalized women in target settings, and (3) ensure the interest of people living in locales where the technology is expected to be implemented and to drive the research agenda.
- The realities of the overall low levels of water and sanitation require redress to improve the health of children in Kenya, Tanzania and Uganda, with equitable access to clean water and sanitation as an important component.

To understand safe water and sanitation in East Africa, we have argued, it is important to consider the contributions of African feminist analysis. Our perspective unveiled inequities in the distribution of these resources and how localized solutions that are driven by women's collaborative work have had an impact in temporarily easing and ameliorating the burden, and we painted a multilayered picture of the lives of women and girls, the predominant providers of water to households. While the summary of lessons from the book is consistent with the advice of female scholars in East African universities, in future work it will be important to examine women activists' views on the matter and to collect sources that come from their organizational websites, news sources, and grey matter in order to identify new areas of inquiry and additional ways to improve access to water and sanitation for the most vulnerable residents of East African communities.

This publication has explored the effects of water and sanitation quality and availability on early childhood morbidity in East Africa from an African feminist sociological perspective. While the individual chapters address specific concerns about women's access to water, failing of sanitation systems, and maternal and child health concerns, comprehensively, we presented a framework that considers the ways that the development industry, neoliberalism, and other aspects of neocolonial relations, gender, class, ethnicity, globalization, and other dimensions of oppression intersect to impact upon the experiences and agency of women and children with accessing clean water and safe sanitation and reducing early childhood morbidity in Kenya, Tanzania, and Uganda. We analyzed recent nationally representative data sets from the Demographic and Health Surveys for each of these countries. On the basis of the African feminist framework, we argued that safe water and sanitation and child health cannot be understood unless socioeconomic, political, and cultural contexts are taken into account. We find that not only are safe water and sanitation in short supply in these countries, but that they also are distributed inequitably, and, further, that the lack of these resources has a deleterious effect on child nutrition. This work enlarged the scope of empirically and theoretically grounded studies within the field of environmental sociology by addressing water and sanitation in an understudied region of the world. Further, this work elicited results that gave rise to useful development effectiveness and child health–related policy recommendations.

Appendix 1

River Basin Model and Decentralization System

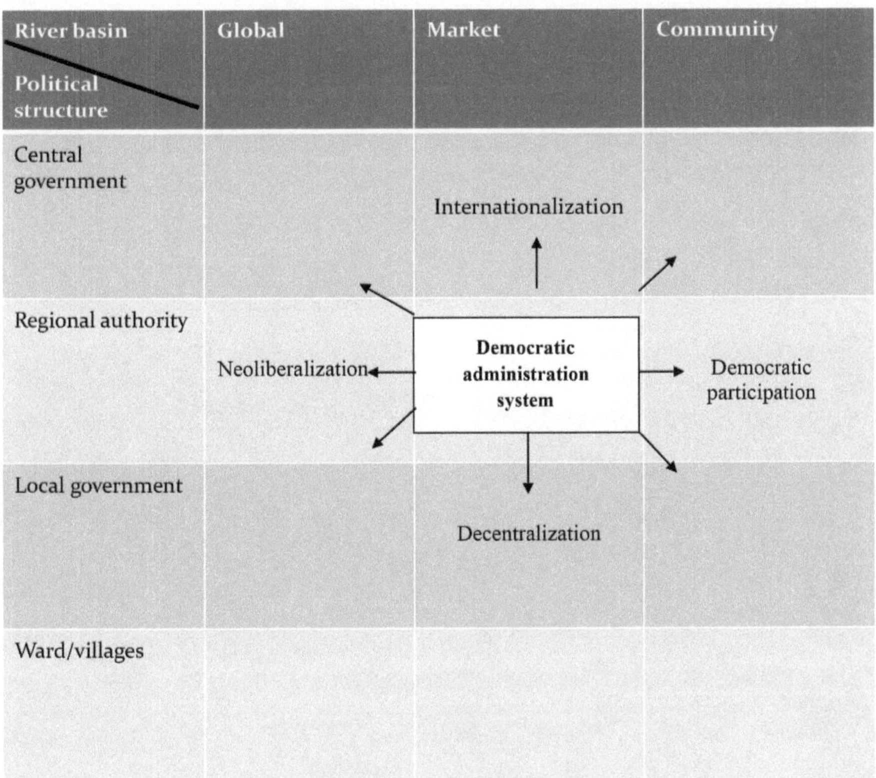

Figure A.1. River Basin Model and Decentralization System

Appendix 2

Population in the Area under Study in Tanzania's Pangani River Basin

Table A.2. Population in the Area under Study in Tanzania's Pangani River Basin

Region	*District*	*Area within Pangani River Basin (km^2)*	*Contribution of Each District to Basin Area (%)*	*Population in 2002*	*Population in Pangani River Basin*	*No. of Households*
Arusha	Arusha	103.51	0.24	282,712	282,712	72,490
	Monduli/ Arumeru	2266.25	5.25	516,814	516,814	112,351
Kilimanjaro	Hai	1224.62	2.84	259,958	129,979	28,884
	Moshi urban	1527.53	3.54	144,336	144,336	35,204
	Moshi rural			402,431	402,431	85,624
	Mwanga	2003.96	4.64	115,620	115,620	24,088
	Rombo	619.93	1.44	246,479	61,620	12,575
	Same	4970.72	11.51	212,325	191,093	39,811
Manyara	Simanjiro	16620.51	38.48	141,676	127,508	29,653
	Kiteto	1290.84	2.99	152,757	15,276	3,182
Tanga	Lushoto	1387.88	3.21	419,970	167,988	35,742
	Korogwe	2974.05	6.89	261,004	261,004	58,001
	Muheza	410.74	0.95	279,423	55,885	12,419
	Pangani	462.86	1.07	44,107	13,232	3,393
	Handeni	4987.64	11.55	249,572	74,872	15,598
	Kilindi			144,359	28,872	5,892
Ocean		7.59	0.02			
Kenya		2333.90	5.40			
	Total area	**43192.54**	**100.0**		**2,589,240**	**574,907**

Source: Turpie, Ngaga, and Karanja (2005).

Appendix 3

Safe Global Water and Sanitation Institute Summit

Program

Held at the Nelson Mandela African Institute of Science and Technology, Arusha, Tanzania
January 30 to February 1, 2013 (with optional activities on February 2)

Wednesday, January 30, Morning
Plenary Session: Climate Change Impact on Water

Registration

Welcome: Burton Mwamila (NMAIST VC)

Remarks/Introduction: Benito Mariñas (University of Illinois at Urbana Champaign [UIUC])

Water–Food–Energy Nexus in the Changing Climate
Zbyszek Kundzewicz

Climate Change/Variability: Definition, Causes and Impacts
Shem Wandiga (UON)

Summit Design/Goals by Benito Mariñas (UIUC)

Session 1: Water–Sanitation Nexus with Energy–Resource Recovery

Introduction (Jörg Drewes)

The State of Water Supply and Wastewater Management in Addis Ababa
Agizew Nigussie, Mengistu Geza, and J. Drewes (AAU + CSM)

Decentralized Management of Wastewater as a Renewable Resource: A Multi-Disciplinary Approach to Sanitation Technology Development
Jeremy Guest and Robinson Ocharo (UIUC + UON)

Clean Household Services: Building Energy and Water?
Tami Bond–Stoves–Safe Air and Water (UIUC)

Tackling Sanitation Problems in Developing Countries: Lessons Learnt from the Use of Constructed Wetland Technology for Domestic Wastewater Treatment
Karoli Njau (NMAIST)

The PSI Program: Community Integration
Nesia Mahenge (PSI) (NGO perspective)

Logical Factors in WaSH Implementation for the Vulnerable Population: Suitability, Convenience, and Patience
Sangam Tiwari (Trussell Technologies)

Community Ownership of Safe Water, Hygiene and Sanitation Practices
Mr. Simon Kajala and Mr. Mika Ayo (Istituto Oikos of East Africa)

Ceramic Water Filtration: From Science to Technology and Applications
Winston Wole Soboyejo (AIST)

Panel Discussion

Thursday, January 31
Opening Ceremony

Arrival of Ministers and Other Dignitaries

Arrival of Prime Minister

Introduction of Summit and Participants
Benito Mariñas (UIUC)

Welcome Remarks by VC of NM-AIST
Burton Mwamila (NM-AIST)

Global Safe Water and Sanitation Issues and Partnerships
Benito Mariñas (UIUC)

Welcome Remarks by the Minister of Communication, Science and Technology
Hon. Prof. Makame Mbarawa (MP)

Opening Address
Hon. Mizengo Pinda (MP), Prime Minister of Tanzania

Vote of Thanks by Chair of NM-AIST Council
Hon. Prof. David Mwakyusa (MP)

Thursday January 31
Session 2: Water/Sanitation Nexus with Health

Introduction (Daniele Lantagne)

Advances in Waterborne Viral Pathogen Control and Sensing
Vincent Madadi, A. Gall, J. Shisler, Y. Lu, B. J. Mariñas, and S. Wandiga (UON + UIUC)

HWTS Successes and Challenges in East Africa
Daniele Lantagne (Tufts)

The SWAP Program in Kenya: Using Local Community Members as Long-Term Change Agents
Alie Eleveld (SWAP)

Impact of Inadequate Sanitation on the Sustainability of Safe Water Systems
J. P. Croue and B. Mariñas (KAUST + UIUC)

Community Perspectives: Addressing Water Quality Challenges in Bondo District
A. J. Rodrigues and S. Wandiga (Bondo + UON)

Experience with the SE2000 Chlorine Generator
Jennifer Foster (PATH)

Safe Filtered Drinking Water in the Home: A Viable Option? Muganyizi Ndyamukama (Winrock)

Multiple-Use Water Services: Moving from Theory to Practice
Muganyizi Ndyamukama and Mary Rernwick (Winrock)

Fluoride Removal/Membrane Technology
Andrea Schäfer and Felix Mtalo (University of Edinburgh + University of Dar es Salaam)

Panel Discussion

Friday, February 1
Session 3: Water/Sanitation Nexus with Nutrition/Food/Environment

Introduction
Water Scarcity and Agriculture: Challenges and Solutions for Africa
Ximing Cai (UIUC)

The Impact of Irrigation on Nutrition, Health and Gender Outcomes
Claudia Ringler (IFPRI)

Microbial Contaminants in Reclaimed Water and Their Potential Impact on Agricultural Irrigation
Peiying Hong (KAUST)

Producing Safe Food Where Irrigation Water is Polluted: From Risk Assessment to Risk Mitigation
Philip Amoah (IWMI)

Water Linking Nutrition, Agriculture and Health
Jeffrey Griffiths (Tufts)

Gender as Social Structure in East Africa and Its Potential Impact on Safe Water
Assata Zerai (UIUC)

Panel Discussion

Session 4: Graduate Student Panel

Introduction (Theresa Vonder Haar)

Partnership Partnerships Bondo District, Kenya
A. Gall (UIUC, UON, BUC)

Emerging Partnerships: Arusha, Tanzania
Lauren Valentino, (UIUC, NMAIST)

Water/Sanitation Nexus with Health: Partnership Action Plan

Water, Nutrition, Food Security, and Environment: Partnership Action Plan

Water–Sanitation Nexus with Energy–Resource Recovery: Partnership Action Plan

Panel Discussion

Closing Remarks

Saturday, February 2 (Optional), Morning or Afternoon
One-Day Safari to Tarangire National Park

Bibliography

Africa Action. 2007. http://www.africaaction.org.

African Population and Health Research Center [APHRC]. 2002. *Population and Health Dynamics in Nairobi's Informal Settlements: Report of the Nairobi Cross-sectional Slums Survey (NCSS) 2000.* Nairobi: APHRC.

African Population and Health Research Center [APHRC]. 2014. *Population and Health Dynamics in Nairobi's Informal Settlements: Report of the Nairobi Cross-sectional Slums Survey (NCSS) 2012*. Nairobi: APHRC.

Agozino, Biko. 1999. "Committed Objectivity in Race, Class, Gender Research." *Quantity and Quality: International Journal of Methodology* 33: 395–410.

Akivaga, S.K., and A.B. Odaga. 1983. *Oral Literature*. Nairobi: Heinemann Educational.

Alexander, M. Jacqui, and Chandra Talpade Mohanty, eds. 1997. *Feminist Genealogies, Colonial Legacies, Democratic Futures*. London: Routledge.

Amadiume, Ifi. 1987. *Male Daughters, Female Husbands: Gender and Sex in an African Society*. London: Zed Books.

Amadiume, Ifi. 1997. Re-Inventing Africa: Matriarchy, Religion, and Culture. London: Zed Books.

Amnesty International. 2010. *Kenya: Insecurity and Indignity: Women's Experiences in the Slums of Nairobi, Kenya.* https://www.amnesty.org/en/documents/AFR32/002/2010/en.

Amoah, Phillip. 2013. "Producing Safe Food Where Irrigantion Water Is Polluted: From Risk Assessment to Risk Migration." Paper presented at the Safe Global Water Summit, Arusha, Tanzania, February 1, 2013.

Ampofo, Akosua Adomako, Josephine Beoku-Betts, Wairimu Ngaruiya Njambi, and Mary Osirim. 2004. "Women's and Gender Studies in English-Speaking Sub-Saharan Africa: A Research in the Social Sciences." *Gender and Society* 18(6): 685–714.

Amuyunzu-Nyamongo, Mary, and Alex Chika Ezeh. 2005. "A Qualitative Assessment of Support Mechanisms in Informal Settlements of Nairobi, Kenya." *Journal of Poverty* 9(3): 89–107.

Angelakis, N. Andreas, and B. Joan Rose. 2014. *Evolution of Sanitation and Wastewater Technologies through the Centuries*. London: IWA Publishing.

Angod, Leila. 2015. "The Unruly Curricula of the Ruling Classes." *Curriculum Inquiry* 45(5): 427–36. DOI: 10.1080/03626784.2015.1103604.

Awino. 2010, June. Personal communication (interview by Brenda N. Sanya).

Bair, Barbara, and Susan Cayleff. 1993. "Foreword," "Preface," and "Introduction." In *Wings of Gauze: Women of Color and the Experience of Health and Illness*, Barbara Bair and Susan Cayleff, eds. Pp. 1–17. Detroit: Wayne State University Press.

Baker, Moses Nelson. 1948. *The Quest for Pure Water; The History of Water Purification from the Earliest Records to the Twentieth Century*. Public Domain, Google-digitized, pp. 1–2. Whitefish, MT: Literary Licensing.

Barham, Elizabeth. 2001. "Ecological Boundaries as Community Boundaries: The Politics of Watershed." *Society and Natural Resources* 14: 181–191.

Barnes, Teresa. 2013. "Pregnancy and Bodies of Knowledge in a South African University." *African Studies Review* 56(1): 1–20. DOI:10.1353/arw.2013.0027.

Beauvoisin, Charlotte. 2013. "The Changing Face of Kampala Slums." *Diary of a Muzungu*. muzungubloguganda.com/2013/03/namuwongo-kampala-slums/#.VP-5Mg4F4pn4.

Beguy, Donatien, Joyce Mumah, and Lindsey Gottschalk. 2014. "Unintended Pregnancies among Young Women Living in Urban Slums: Evidence from a Prospective Study in Nairobi City, Kenya." *Plos ONE* 9(7): 1–10.

Behrendt, Stephen D. 2008. Seasonality in the Trans-Atlantic Slave Trade. https://scholar.google.com/scholar?um=1&ie=UTF-8&lr&q=related:BxtM-5rD7NU89M:scholar.google.com.

Berlant, L.G. 2011. *Cruel Optimism*. Durham, NC: Duke University Press.

Biswas, Asit K. 2008. "Integrated Water Resources Management: Is It Working?" *Water Resources Development* 24(1): 5–22.

Blanton, Elizabeth, N. Wilhelm, C. O'Reilly, E. Muhonja, S. Karoki, M. Ope, D. Langat, J. Omolo, N. Wamola, J. Oundo, R. Hoekstra, T. Ayers, K. De Cock, R. Breiman, E. Mintz, and D. Lantagne. 2015. "A Rapid Assessment of Drinking Water Quality in Informal Settlements after a Cholera Outbreak in Nairobi, Kenya." *Journal of Water and Health* 13(3): 714–725.

Bloomfield, Sally, R. Stanwell-Smith, R.W.R. Crevel, and J. Pickup. 2006. "Too Clean, or Not Too Clean: The Hygiene Hypothesis and Home Hygiene." *Clinical and Experimental Allergy* 36(4): 402–25.

Bond, Tami. 2013. "Clean Household Services: Building Energy and Water?" Paper presented at the Safe Global Water Summit, Arusha, Tanzania, February 1, 2013.

Boserup, Ester. 1970. *Woman's Role in Economic Development*. London: George Allen and Unwin.

Bouckaert, Peter. 1999. *Hostile to Democracy: The Movement System and Political Repression in Uganda Human Right Watch World Report*. https://www.hrw.org/reports/1999/uganda/Uganweb-11.htm.

Breiman, Robert F., Leonard Cosmas, M. Kariuki Njenga, John Williamson, Joshua A. Mott, Mark A. Katz, Dean D. Erdman, Eileen Schneider, M. Steven Oberste, John C. Neatherlin, Henry Njuguna, Daniel M. Ondari, Kennedy Odero, George

O. Okoth, Beatrice Olack, Newton Wamola, Joel M. Montgomery, Barry S. Fields, and Daniel R. Feikin. 2015. "Severe Acute Respiratory Infection in Children in a Densely Populated Urban Slum in Kenya, 2007–2011." *BMC Infectious Diseases* 15(1): 1–11.

Brown, Elsa Barkley. 1995. "'What Has Happened Here': The Politics of Difference in Women's History and Feminist Politics." In *We Specialize in the Wholly Impossible: A Reader in Black Women's History*, Darlene Clark Hine, Wilma King, and Linda Reed, eds. Pp. 39–54. Brooklyn: Carlson Publishing.

Brown, Rebecca. 2010. "Unequal Burden: Water Privatization and Women's Human Rights in Tanzania." *Gender and Development* 18(1): 59–67.

Bryman, Alan. 2004. *Social Research Methods*. Oxford: Oxford University Press.

Cai, Ximing. 2013. "Introduction-Nutrition/Food/Environment." Paper presented at the Safe Global Water Summit, Arusha, Tanzania, February 1, 2013.

Cairncross, Sandy, and Vivian Valdmanis. 2006. "Water Supply, Sanitation, and Hygiene Promotion." In D.T. Jamison, J.G. Breman, A.R. Measham, G. Alleyne, M. Claeson, D.B. Evans, P. Jha, A. Mills, and P. Musgrove, eds. *Disease Control Priorities in Developing Countries*, 2nd ed. Pp. 771–92. Washington, DC: World Bank.

Caldwell, John C. 1985. "The Social Repercussions of Colonial Rule: Demographic Aspects." In UNESCO *General History of Africa*, Volume 7: *Africa under Colonial Domination*. A. Adu Boahen, ed. Pp. 458-486. Heinemann: London.

Campbell, Horace. 2003. *Reclaiming Zimbabwe: The Exhaustion of the Patriarchal Model of Liberation*. Claremont, South Africa: David Philip.

Campbell, James. 1871. *The Advanced Book of Reading Lessons*. Canadian Series of School Books. Toronto: James Campbell and Sons.

Caulfield, Laura E., Stephanie A. Richard, and Robert E. Black. 2004. "Undernutrition as an Underlying Cause of Malaria Morbidity and Mortality in Children Less than Five Years Old." *American Journal of Tropical Medicine* 71(2 Suppl): 55–63.

Center for Reproductive Rights. 2007. *Failure to Deliver: Violations of Women's Human Rights in Kenyan Health Facilities*. New York, Nairobi: Center for Reproductive Rights. https://www.reproductiverights.org/sites/crr.civicactions.net/files/documents/pub_bo_failuretodeliver.pdf.

Charmaz, Kathy. 1991. *Good Days, Bad Days: The Self and Chronic Illness in Time*. New Brunswick, NJ: Rutgers University Press.

Charmaz, Kathy, and Debora A. Paterniti. 1999. "Introduction." In *Health, Illness and Healing: Society, Social Context, and Self*, Kathy Charmaz and Debora A. Paterniti, eds. Los Angeles: Roxbury Publishing.

Chepyator-Thomson, Jepkorir Rose, ed. 2005. *African Women and Globalization: Dawn of the 21st Century*. Trenton, NJ: Africa World Press.

Christensen, J. 2015. "Devices of Wonder." *Virginia Quarterly Review* 91(3): 52–57.

Collins, Patricia Hill. 1986. "Learning from the Outsider Within: The Sociological Significance of Black Feminist Thought." *Social Problems* 33(6): S14–S32. DOI: 10.2307/800672.

Collins, Patricia Hill. 1990. *Black Feminist Thought: Knowledge, Consciousness, and the Politics of Empowerment*, 2nd ed. Boston: Unwin Hyman.

Collins, Patricia Hill. 1998. *Fighting Words: Black Women and the Search for Justice.* Minneapolis: University of Minnesota Press.

Conrad, Peter, and Valerie Leiter. 2003. "Introduction." In *Health and Health Care as Social Problems*, Peter Conrad and Valerie Leiter, eds. Pp. 1–6. Lanham, MD: Rowman & Littlefield.

Croue, Jean-Philippe, and Benito Marinas. 2013. "Impact of Inadequate Sanitation Sustainability of Safe Water Systems." Paper presented at the Safe Global Water Summit, Arusha, Tanzania, February 1.

Daily Monitor. 2012, May 24. *Politics of Migrant Labour and Uneven Development in Uganda's Colonial-Era.* http://www.monitor.co.ug/SpecialReports/ugandaat50/-/1370466/1412250/-/view/printVersion/-/rc2ajr/-/index.html.

Davis, Angela Y. 1981. *Women, Race, and Class.* New York: Random House.

Davis, Angela Y. 1990. *Women, Culture, and Politics.* New York: Vintage Books.

Decker, Alicia. 2010. "Idi Amin's Dirty War: Subversion, Sabotage, and the Battle to Keep Uganda Clean, 1971–1979." *International Journal of African Historical Studies* 43(3): 489–513.

Demographic and Health Surveys [DHS]. 2011. www.measuredhs.com/start.cfm.

Desai, Karishma. 2016. "Teaching the Third World Girl: Girl Rising as a Precarious Curriculum of Empathy." *Curriculum Inquiry* 46(3): 248–64. DOI: 10.1080/03626784.2016.1173510.

Diamond, Timothy. 1992. *Making Gray Gold: Narratives of Nursing Home Care.* Chicago: University of Chicago Press.

Dreibelbis, R., M.C. Freeman, L.E. Greene, S. Saboori, and R. Rheingans. 2014. "The Impact of School Water, Sanitation, and Hygiene Interventions on the Health of Younger Siblings of Pupils: A Cluster-Randomized Trial in Kenya." *American Journal of Public Health* 104(1): e91–e97.

Drewes, Jorg. 2013. "Introduction: Energy/Resource Nexus." Paper presented at the Safe Global Water Summit, Arusha, Tanzania, February 1, 2013.

Du Bois, William E.B. 1965. {1947}. *The World and Africa.* New York: International Publishers.

Durkheim, Emile. 1951. *Suicide: A Study in Sociology.* J. Spaulding and G. Simpson, trans. New York: Free Press.

East African Community (EAC). 2001. www.eac.int.

East African Community (EAC). 2016. *East African Community (EAC) Vision* 2050. www.eac.int/sites/default/files/docs/eac_vision_2050-_web.pdf.

Eleveld, Alie. 2013. *The SWAP Program in Kenya: Using Local Community Members as Long-Term Change Agents.* Paper presented at the Safe Global Water Summit, Arusha, Tanzania, February 1.

Ellis, Frank, and N. Mdoe. 2003. "Rural Livelihoods and Poverty Reduction in Tanzania." *World Development* 40: 1367–1384.

Encyclopedia Britannica Online. https://www.britannica.com/technology/noria.

Fall, Ibrahima-Soce. 2016. "Outbreaks and Emergencies." *Bulletin Regional Office of Africa* 6(4): 1–10.

Fanon, Frantz. 1968. *The Wretched of the Earth.* New York: Grove.

Federici, Silvia. 2004. *Caliban and the Witch: Women, the Body and Primitive Accumulation*. Brooklyn: Autonomedia.

Foster, Jennifer. 2013. "Africa User Research in Water Sanitation." Paper presented at the Safe Global Water Summit, Arusha, Tanzania, February 1.

Freeman, Carla. 2001. "Is Local: Global as Feminine: Masculine? Rethinking the Gender of Globalization." *Signs* 26: 1007–1037.

Friedman J.F., A.M. Kwena, L.B. Mirel, S.K. Kariuki, D.J. Terlouw, P.A. Phillips-Howard, W.A. Hawley, B.L. Nahlen, Y.P. Shi, and F.O. ter Kuile. 2005. "Malaria and Nutritional Status among Pre-School Children: Results from Cross-Sectional Surveys in Western Kenya." *American Journal of Tropical Medicine and Hygiene* 73: 698–704.

Fuller, James A., Thomas Clasen, Marieke Heijnen, and Joseph N.S. Eisenberg. 2014. "Shared Sanitation and the Prevalence of Diarrhea in Young Children: Evidence from 51 Countries, 2001–2011."*American Journal of Tropical Medicine and Hygiene* 91(1): 173–180. DOI: 10.4269/ajtmh.13-0503.

Gachukia, E., and S.K. Akivaga. 1978. *Teaching of African Literature in Schools*. Nairobi, London: Kenya Literature Bureau.

Gaidzanwa, Rudo B. 1997. "Gender Analysis in the Field of Education: A Zimbabwean Example." In *Engendering African Social Sciences*, Ayesha Imam, Amina Mama, and Fatou Sow, eds. Pp. 271–296. Dakar: CODESRIA.

Gordon, Lewis. 2006. *An Introduction to African Philosophy*. Cambridge: Cambridge University Press.

Government of the Republic of Kenya. 2007. *Vision 2030*. www.vision2030.go.ke.

Government of the Republic of Kenya. 2010. *Kenya Health Facilities: Nyawara Health Centre*. http://www.ehealth.or.ke/facilities/facility.aspx?fas=13947.

Green, Elliott. 2010a. "Patronage, District Creation and Reform in Uganda." *Studies in Comparative International Development* 45(1): 83–103.

Green, Elliott. 2010b. "Ethnicity and Nationhood in Precolonial Africa: The Case of Buganda." *Nationalism and Ethnic Politics* 16(1): 1–21.

Griffiths, Jeffrey. 2013. "Water Linking Nutrition, Agriculture and Health." Paper presented at the Safe Global Water Summit, Arusha, Tanzania, February 1.

Guest, Jeremy. 2013. "Decentralized Management of Wastewater as a Renewable Resource: A Multi-Disciplinary Approach to Sanitation Technology Development." Paper presented at the Safe Global Water Summit, Arusha, Tanzania, February 1, 2013.

Guicheng, Zhang et al. 2005. Household Hygiene. *Pediatric Allergy & Immunology* 16(7): 587–92.

Hair, Joseph F. Jr., William C. Black, J. Barry Babin, Rolph E. Anderson, and Ronald L. Tatham. 2006. *Multivariate Data Analysis, 6th ed*. Upper Saddle River, NJ: Pearson Education.

Hamel, M.J., K. Adazu, D. Obor, M. Sewe, J. Vulule, J.M. Williamson, L. Slutsker, D.R. Felkin, and K.F. Laserson. 2011. "A Reversal in Reductions of Child Mortality in Western Kenya, 2003–2009." *American Journal of Tropical Medicine and Hygiene* 85: 597–605. DOI: 10.4269/ajtmh.2011.10-0678.

Harding, Sandra, ed. 1987. "Introduction" and "Conclusion." In *Feminism and Methodology*. Bloomington: Indiana University Press.

Harding, Sandra, and Kathryn Norberg. 2005. "New Feminist Approaches to Social Science Methodologies: An Introduction." *Signs* 30: 2009–2015.

Harris, Julie. n.d. "Getting Ahead in the Slums of Kampala." *Concern Worldwide*. www.concern.net/where-we-work/africa/uganda/helping-women-get-ahead-slums-kampala.

Harrison, Faye. 2016. Personal communication.

Hawkesworth, M.E. 2006. *Globalization and Feminist Activism*. Lanham, MD: Rowman & Littlefield.

Headey, D., and K. Hirvonen. 2016. "Is Exposure to Poultry Harmful to Child Nutrition? An Observational Analysis for Rural Ethiopia." *PLoS ONE* 1(8): 1–16.

Henderson, Loren, Assata Zerai, and Rebecca Morrow. 2017. "Intimate Partner Violence and HIV Status among Ever-Married and Cohabiting Zimbabwean Women: An Examination of Partners' Traits." *African Journal of Reproductive Health* 21(4). (December 2017 Edition).

Henderson, Shirley. 2004. "Introduction to Health within SADC." In *The Gender Perspective: Innovations in Economy, Organizations, and Health within Southern African Development Community (SADC).* Ingelore Welpe, Britta Thege, and Shirley Henderson, eds. Pp. 304–313. New York: P. Lang.

Hoag, Heather J. 2006. "Transplanting the TVA? International Contributions to Postwar River Development in Tanzania." *Comparative Technology Transfer and Society* 4(3): 247–68.

Hong, Peiying. 2013. "Microbial Contaminants in Reclaimed Water and Their Potential Impact on Agricultural Irrigation." Paper presented at the Safe Global Water Summit, Arusha, Tanzania, February 1.

Hooper, M. 2012. "Lessons from Mobilisation around Slum Evictions in Tanzania." *Revista Migraciones Forzadas* 41: 47.

Human Rights Watch. 2010. Toxic Toil: Child Labor and Mercury Exposure in Tanzania's Small-Scale Gold Mines. https://www.hrw.org/report/2013/08/28/toxic-toil/child-labor-and-mercury-exposure-tanzanias-small-scale-gold-mines.

Humphrey, Jean H. 2009. "Child Undernutrition, Tropical Enteropathy, Toilets, and Handwashing." *Lancet* 374: 1032–1035. DOI 10.1016/S0140-6736(09)60950-8.

ICF International. 2012. The DHS Program STATcompiler. www.statcompiler.com.

Imam, Ayesha M., and Amina Mama. 1994. "Role of Academics in Limiting and Expanding Academic Freedom." In *Academic Freedom in Africa.* Mahmood Mamdani and Mamadou Diouf, eds. Pp. 73–107. Dakar: CODESRIA.

Imam, Ayesha M., Amina Mama, and Fatou Sow, eds. 1997. *Engendering African Social Sciences*. Dakar: CODESRIA.

Jafri, B. 2017. Ongoing Colonial Violence in Settler States. *Lateral* 6(1). DOI: 10.251 58/16.1.7.

Jansz, Shamila, and Jane Wilbur. 2013. "Water Supply and Sanitation, Water Aid." www.wateraid.org/~/media/Publications/Women-and-WASH.pdf.

Kajala, Simon and Mika Ayo. 2013. "Community Ownership of Safe Water, Hygiene, and Sanitation Practice." Paper presented at the Safe Global Water Summit, Arusha, Tanzania, February 1.

Kanbur, Ravi, ed. 2001. *Q-Squared: Qualitative and Quantitative Methods of Poverty Appraisal*. New Delhi: Permanent Black.

Kauanui, J.K. 2016. "'A Structure, Not an Event': Settler Colonialism and Enduring Indigeneity." *Lateral* 5(1). DOI: 10.25158/15.1.7.

Katukiza, A.Y., M. Ronteltap, A. Oleja, C.B. Niwagaba, F. Kansiime, and P.N. Lens. 2010. "Selection of Sustainable Sanitation Technologies for Urban Slums: A Case of Bwaise III in Kampala, Uganda." *Science of the Total Environment* 409: 52–62.

Kemper, Karin E., William Blomquist, and Ariel Dinar, eds. 2007. *Integrated River Basin Management through Decentralization*. Berlin: Springer.

Kenya National Bureau of Statistics. 2012. 2009 Kenya Population Census, *Analytical Report on Housing Conditions, Amenities and Household Assets*, Volume XI.

Kenya National Bureau of Statistics [KNBS] and ICF Macro. 2010. *Kenya Demographic and Health Survey: Country Report 2008–09*. Calverton, MD: KNBS and ICF Macro.

Kenya National Bureau of Statistics [KNBS] and ICF Macro. 2014. *Kenya Demographic and Health Survey*. [Dataset]. Calverton, MD: KNBS and ICF Macro.

Kenya National Bureau of Statistics [KNBS] and ICF Macro. 2014. *Kenya Demographic and Health Survey 2014*. Rockville, MD, USA: Kenya National Bureau of Statistics, Ministry of Health/Kenya, National AIDS Control Council/Kenya, Kenya Medical Research Institute, National Council for Population and Development/Kenya, and ICF International.

Kenya National Bureau of Statistics, Ministry of Health/Kenya, National AIDS Control Council/Kenya, Kenya Medical Research Institute, National Council for Population and Development/Kenya, and ICF International, 2015. *Kenya Demographic and Health Survey: Country Report 2014.* Calverton, MD: KNBS and ICF Macro.

Kenya Vision 2030. 2016. www.vision2030.g0.ke/about-vision-2030.

Kimeker, Koipano, and Felistus Gilai. 2014. *What It Means to Be a Girl in My Village*. Poem showcased at Girls Speak Out, United Nations Day of the Girl, October 2014. https://www.one.org/us/2015/09/16/what-it-means-to-be-a-girl-in-my-village.

Klugman, Barbara. 2011. "Effective Social Justice Advocacy: A Theory-of-Change Framework for Assessing Progress." *Reproductive Health Matters* 19(38): 146–62.

Korpe, Poonum S., and William A. Petri, Jr. 2012. "Environmental Enteropathy: Critical Implications of a Poorly Understood Condition." *Trends in Molecular Medicine* 18: 328–36. DOI: 10.1016/j.molmed.2012.04.007.

Krieger, Nancy, and Elizabeth Fee. 1994. "Man-Made Medicine and Women's Health: The Biopolitics of Sex/Gender and Race/Ethnicity." *International Journal of Health Services* 24: 265–83.

Kundzewicz, Zbyszek. 2013. "Water–Food–Energy Nexus in the Changing Climate." Presentation at the Safe Global Water Summit, Arusha, Tanzania, Jan. 30–Feb. 1.

Kwiringira, Japheth, Peter Atekyereza, Charles Niwagaba and Isabel Günther. 2014. "Descending the Sanitation Ladder in Urban Uganda: Evidence from Kampala Slums." *Bio Med Central (BMC) Public Health* 14: 624.

Kwiringira, Japheth, Peter Atekyereza, Charles Niwagaba, Robert Kabumbuli, Charles Rwabukwali, Robinah Kulabako, and Isabel Günther. 2016. "Seasonal

Variations and Shared Latrine Cleaning Practices in the Slums of Kampala City, Uganda." *Bio Med Central (BMC) Public Health* 16: 361.

Kyobutung, Catherine, Abdhalah Kasiira Ziraba, Alex Ezeh, and Yazoumé Yé. 2008. "The Burden of Disease Profile of Residents of Nairobi's Slums: Results from a Demographic Surveillance System." *Population Health Metrics* 6(1): 1–8. DOI: 10.1186/1478-7954-6-1.

Lall, Somik. 2015 *Planning for Uganda's Urbanization Inclusive Growth Policy Note 4*. World Bank Group. siteresources.worldbank.org/INTUGANDA/Resources/uganda-urbanization-full-policy-note.pdf.

Langdon, Steve. 1974. "The Political Economy of Dependence: Note toward Analysis of Multinational Corporations in Kenya." *Journal of East African Research and Development* 4: 123–59.

Lantagne, Daniele. 2013. "Introduction–Health Nexus." Paper presented at the Safe Global Water Summit, Arusha, Tanzania, February 1.

Legros, D., M. McCormick, C. Mugero, M. Skinnider, D.D. Bek'Obita, and S.I. Okware. 2000. "Epidemiology of Cholera Outbreak in Kampala, Uganda." *East African Medical Journal* 77(7): 347–49.

Lein, Haakon. 2004. "Managing the Water of Kilimanjaro: Irrigation, Peasants and Hydropower Development." *Geo Journal* 61(2): 155–62.

Lein, Haakon, and Mattias Tagseth. 2009. "Tanzanian Water Policy Reforms: Between Principles and Practical Applications." *Water Policy* 11(2): 203–20.

Levira, Beda Modest. 2016. *Water Points Situation in the Kilombero District and Rehabilitation Plan.* blog.msabi.org/2016/03/water-points-situation-in-kilombero_14.html.

Lim, Stephen S (with >100 GBD 2015 SDG Collaborators). 2016. "Measuring the Health-Related Sustainable Development Goals in 188 Countries: A Baseline Analysis from the Global Burden of Disease Study 2015." *Lancet* 388 (10053): 1813–50.

Loevinsohn, M., L. Mehta, K. Cuming, A. Nicol, O. Cumming, and J.H.J. Ensink. 2015. "The Cost of a Knowledge Silo: A Systematic Re-Review of Water, Sanitation and Hygiene Interventions." *Health Policy and Planning* 30(5): 660–74.

Lorde, Audre. 1984. "Age, Race, Class, and Sex: Women Defining Difference." In *Sister Outsider*, Audre Lorde, ed. Pp. 114–23. Trumansburg, NY: Crossing Press.

Macharia, K. 2017. *The Development Imaginary: Tracks*. https://thenewinquiry.com/blogs/wiathi/the-development-imaginary-tracks.

Machiwa, Praxeda K. 2003. "Water Quality Management and Sustainability: The Experience of Lake Victoria Environmental Management Project." *Physics and Chemistry of the Earth*, Parts A/B/C. 28: 1111–1115. DOI: 10.1016/j.pce.2003.08.032.

Mackintosh, Maureen, and Paula Tibandebage. 2006. "Gender and Health Sector Reform: Analytic Perspectives on African Experience." In *Gender and Social Policy in a Global Context: Uncovering the Gendered Structure of "The Social."* S. Razavi and S. Hassin, eds. Pp. 237–57. Basingstoke, England: Palgrave Macmillan.

MacPherson, Stewart. 1982. *Social Policy in the Third World.* Brighton, UK: Wheatsheaf.

Madadi, Vincent, Aimee Gall, Joanna Shisler, Y. Lu, Benito Marinas, and Shem O. Wandiga. 2013. "Advances in Waterborne Viral Pathogen Control and Sensing." Paper presented at the Safe Global Water Summit, Arusha, Tanzania, February 1.

Magigi, W., and B. Majani. 2006. "Community Involvement in Land Regularization for Informal Settlements in Tanzania: A Strategy for Enhancing Security of Tenure in Residential Neighborhoods." *Habitat International* 30(4): 1066–81.

Mahenge, Nesia. 2013. "Household Water Treatment for Prevention of Diarrhea Disease in Tanzania." Paper presented at the Safe Global Water Summit, Arusha, Tanzania, February 1.

Makoka, Donald, and Peninah Kinya Masibo. 2015. "Is There a Threshold Level of Maternal Education Sufficient to Reduce Child Undernutrition? Evidence from Malawi, Tanzania and Zimbabwe." *BioMed Central Pediatrics* 15(96): 1–10. DOI: 10.1186/s12887-015-0406-8.

Malipula, Mariso. 2014. "Depoliticized Ethnicity in Tanzania: A Structural and Historical Narrative." *Afrika Focus* 27(2): 49–70.

Mama, Amina. 2000. "Strengthening Civil Society: Participatory Action Research in Militarized State." *Development in Practice* 10: 59–70.

Mama, Amina. 2002. "Editorial." *Feminist Africa: Intellectual Politics* 1: 150.

Mama, Amina. 2011. "The Challenges of Feminism: Gender, Ethics and Responsible Academic Freedom in African Universities." *Journal of Higher Education in Africa* 9(2): 1–23.

Mariwah, S., K. Hampshire, and A. Kasim. 2012. "The Impact of Gender and Physical Environment on the Handwashing Behaviour of University Students in Ghana." *Tropical Medicine and International Health* 17(4): 447–54.

Martin, William G., and Michael O. West. 1999. "The Ascent, Triumph, and Disintegration of the Africanist Enterprise, U.S.A." In *Out of One, Many Africas: Reconstructing the Study and Meaning of Africa.* William G. Martin and Michael O. West, eds. Pp. 85–122. Chicago, Urbana: University of Illinois Press.

Matanda, D.J., M.B. Mittelmark, and D.M.D. Kigaru. 2014. "Child Undernutrition in Kenya: Trend Analyses from 1993 to 2008–09." *BMC Pediatrics* 14: 5. DOI: 10.1186/1471-2431-14-5.

Matubaazi, Enoch. 2006. "A Day in Katanga." *U.G. Pulse*. www.ugpulse.com/travel-and-tourism/a-day-in-katanga/487/ug.aspx.

Mbilinyi, Dorothy A. 1996. "Women and Gender Relations in School Textbooks." In *Gender Relations and Women's Images in the Media,* Dorothy A.S. Mbilinyi and Cuthbert K. Omari, eds. Pp. 90–99. Dar es Salaam: Dar es Salaam University Press.

Mbuya, M.N.N., and J.H. Humphrey. 2016. "Preventing Environmental Enteric Dysfunction through Improved Water, Sanitation and Hygiene: An Opportunity for Stunting Reduction in Developing Countries." *Maternal and Child Nutrition* 12: 106–20.

McKinsey Global Institute. September 2015. *The Power of Parity: How Advancing Women's Equality Can Add $12 Trillion to Global Growth.* www.mckinsey.com/mgi.

Meilicke, G., A. Weissenborn, W. Biederbick, and C. Bartels. 2008. "Fighting the Flu with Soap and Water: Hand Washing as an Infection Control Recommendation to the Population—7 Hypotheses from a Qualitative Study About Hygiene, Flu and Pandemic." *Bundesgesundheitsblatt–Gesundheitsforschung–Gesundheitsschutz* 51(11): 1273–79.

Millennium Villages. 2010. *Millennium Village in Sauri, Kenya.* millenniumvillages.org/the-villages/sauri-kenya.

Ministry of Finance, Planning and Economic Development. 2013. *Millennium Development Goals Report for Uganda 2013: Drivers of MDG Progress in Uganda and Implications for the Post-2015 Development Agenda.* Kampala: Ministry of Finance, Planning and Economic Development.

Ministry of Health, Community Development, Gender, Elderly and Children (MoHCDGEC) [Tanzania Mainland]; Ministry of Health (MoH) [Zanzibar]; National Bureau of Statistics (NBS); Office of the Chief Government Statistician (OCGS); and ICF. 2016. *Tanzania Demographic and Health Survey and Malaria Indicator Survey (TDHS-MIS) 2015–16.* Dar es Salaam, Tanzania, and Rockville, Maryland: MoHCDGEC, MoH, NBS, OCGS, and ICF.

Ministry of Planning and National Development, the Government of Kenya, and the United Nations, Kenya. 2003. *Kenya MDGs Progress Report. Nairobi Urban Sector Profile.* Nairobi: United Nations Human Settlements Programme.

Ministry of State for Planning, National Development and Vision 2030. 2008. "Launching of Kenya Vision 2030 Speech by His Excellency Hon. Mwai Kibaki, CGH, MP."

Molden, D., ed. 2007. *Water for Life, Water for Good: A Comprehensive Assessment of Water Management in Agriculture.* International Water Management Institute. Columbo and Earthscan: London.

Molyneux, Maxine. 2006. "Mothers at the Service of the New Poverty Agenda: The PROGRESA/Opurtunidades Programme in Mexico." In *Gender and Social Policy in a Global Context: Uncovering the Gendered Structure of "The Social,"* S. Razavi and S. Hassin, eds. Pp. 43–67. Basingstoke, England: Palgrave Macmillan.

Mozans, H. J. 1913. "Women in Science: With an Introductory Chapter on Woman's Long Struggle for Things of the Mind." New York, London: D. Appleton.

Mudege, Netsayi, and Eliya Zulu. 2011. "Discourses of Illegality and Exclusion: When Water Access Matters." *Global Public Health* 6(3): 221–33.

Mugo, Micere Githae. 1991. *African Orature and Human Rights.* Roma, Lesotho: Institute of Southern African Studies, National University of Lesotho.

Mutibwa, Phares. 1992. *Uganda Since Independence: A Story of Unfulfilled Hopes.* Trenton, NJ: Africa World Press.

Muyambo, T., and R.S. Maposa. 2014. "Linking Culture and Water Technology in Zimbabwe: Reflections on Ndau Experiences and Implications for Climate Change." *Journal of African Studies and Development* 6(2), 22–28. DOI: 10.5897/JASD2013.0266.

Mwanza, Allast M., ed. 1992. *Structural Adjustment Programmes in SADC: Experiences and Lessons from Malawi, Tanzania, Zambia, and Zimbabwe.* Harare: SAPES.

National Bureau of Statistics/Tanzania and Macro International. 2000. *Tanzania Reproductive and Child Health Survey 1999*. Calverton, MD: National Bureau of Statistics/Tanzania and Macro International.

National Bureau of Statistics (NBS) [Tanzania] and ICF Macro. 2011. *Tanzania Demographic and Health Survey Country Report 2010. Dar es Salaam, Tanzania: NBS and ICF Macro.*

Ndiritu, Nelson, Jacinta Ndambuki, and James Onyango. 2016. "Promoting Post-Conflict Peaceful Co-Existence in Multi-Ethnic Communities: Lessons from Internally Displaced Persons in Kenya." *Africology: The Journal of Pan African Studies* 9(10): 122–40.

Ngare, D.K., and J.N. Muttunga 1999. "Prevalence of Malnutrition in Kenya." *East African Medical Journal* 76(7): 376–80.

Nigussie, Agizew, Mengistu Geza, and Jorg Drewes. 2013. "State of Water Supply and Wastewater Management in Addis Ababa." Paper presented at the Safe Global Water Summit, Arusha, Tanzania, February 1.

Njau, Karoli. 2013. "Tackling Sanitation Problems in Developing Countries: Lessons Learnt from the Use of Constructed Wetlands Technology for Domestic Waste Water Treatment." Paper presented at the Safe Global Water Summit, Arusha, Tanzania, February 1.

Nkrumah, Kwame. 1963. *Africa Must Unite.* New York: Praejer.

Nyong'o, Anyang'. 1988. "Industrial Possibility and Historical Limitations." In *Industrialization in Kenya: In Search of a Strategy*, Peter E. Coughlin and Gerrishon K. Ikiara, eds. Pp. 17–25. Nairobi: East African Educational Publishers.

Nyong'o, Anyang'. 2007. *A Leap into the Future: A Vision for Kenya's Socio-Political and Economic Transformation*. Nairobi: African Research and Resource Forum.

Nzegwu, N. 2004. "Feminism and Africa: Impact and Limits of the Metaphysics of Gender." *A Companion to African Philosophy*, Kwasi Wiredu, ed. Pp. 560–69. Cambridge, MA: Blackwell Publishing.

Ogot, Bethwell A. 1967. *History of the Southern Luo*. Nairobi: East African Publishing.

Ogwang, Joel. 2013. "Slums Present a Fierce Challenge to Uganda's Urbanisation Effort." *Vision*. www.newvision.co.ug/news/640621-slums-present-a-fierce-challenge-to-uganda-s-urbanisation-effort.html.

Okech, Awino. 2011. "Alternative Discourses: A Feminist Approach to Re-Thinking Security." In *Women and Security Governance in Africa*, Funmi Olonisakin and Awino Okech, eds. Pp. 49–68. Cape Town: Pambazuka Press.

Okia, Opolot. 2012. *Communal Labor in Colonial Kenya: The Legitimization of Coercion, 1912–1930*. New York: Palgrave Macmillan.

Olack, B., D.R. Feikin, L.O. Cosmas, K.O. Odero, G.O. Okoth, J.M. Montgomery, and R.F. Breiman. 2014. "Mortality Trends Observed in Population-Based Surveillance of an Urban Slum Settlement, Kibera, Kenya, 2007–2010." *Plos ONE* 9(1): 1–6.

Osirim, Mary J. 2003. "Crisis in the State and the Family: Violence Against Women in Zimbabwe." *African Studies Quarterly* 7(2, 3): 153–69.

Oyěwùmí, Oyèrónkẹ́. 1997. *The Invention of Women: Making an African Sense of Western Gender Discourses*. Minneapolis: University of Minnesota Press.

Oyěwùmí, Oyèrónkẹ́, ed. 2003. *African Women and Feminism: Reflecting on the Politics of Sisterhood.* Trenton, NJ: Africa World Press.

Oyěwùmí, Oyèrónkẹ́, ed. 2005. *African Gender Studies: Theoretical Questions and Conceptual Issues*. New York: Palgrave MacMillan.

Pallant, Jennifer. 2003. *SPSS Survival Manual. A Step by Step Guide to Data Analysis Using SPSS for Windows (Versions 10 and 11).* Maidenhead, PA: Open University Press.

Penrose, K., M.C. de Castro, J. Werema, and E.T. Ryan. 2010. Informal Urban Settlements and Cholera Risk in Dar es Salaam, Tanzania. *Plos Neglected Tropical Diseases* 4(3): 1–11.

PMA. 2015. Uganda. Performance Monitoring and Accountability 2020. http://pma2020.org/sites/default/files/SDG-Indicator%20brief-v16-2016.05.18.pdf.

Prendergast, A.J., and J.H. Humphrey. 2015. *Stunting Persists Despite Optimal Feeding: Are Toilets Part of the Solution?* Nestle Nutrition Institute Workshop Series 81: 99–110. DOI:10.1159/000365807.

Prieto, Laura R. 2010. "'Stepmother America': The Woman's Board of Missions in the Philippines, 1902–1930." In *Competing Kingdoms: Women, Mission, Nation, and the American Protestant Empire, 1812–1960*, Barbara Reeves-Ellington, Kathryn Kish Sklar, and Connie A. Shemo, eds. Pp. 342–66. Durham, NC: Duke University Press.

Puri, J. 2004. *Encountering Nationalism*. Malden, MA: Blackwell.

Qunta, Christine, ed. 1987. *Women in Southern Africa*. Johannesburg: Skotaville.

Rabaka, Reiland. 2010. *Epistemic Apartheid: W.E.B. Du Bois and the Disciplinary Decadence of Sociology.* Lanham, MD: Lexington.

Razack, S. 2002. *Race, Space, and the Law: Unmapping a White Settler Society.* Toronto: Between the Lines.

Razack, S. 2004. *Dark Threats and White Knights: The Somalia Affair, Peacekeeping, and the New Imperialism.* Toronto: University of Toronto Press.

Reid, Richard. 2014. "Ghosts in the Academy: Historians and Historical Consciousness in the Making of Modern Uganda." *Comparative Studies in Society and History.* 56(2): 351–80.

Republic of Kenya, Ministry of Education, Science and Technology. 2015. *National Education Sector Plan. Volume One: Basic Education Programme Rationale and Approach 2013–2018.* www.education.go.ke.

Reuters. 2011. "Tanzania Power Cuts Worsen after Drought." Thomson Reuters. http://af.reuters.com/article/investingNews/idAFJOE71E0HR20110215.

Ring, J., U. Krämer, and H. Behrendt. 2004. "A Critical Approach to the Hygiene Hypothesis." *Clinical and Experimental Allergy Reviews* 4: 40–44.

Ringer, Claudia. 2013. "Impact of Irrigation on Nutrition, Health and Gender Outcomes." Paper presented at the Safe Global Water Summit, Arusha, Tanzania, February 1, 2013.

Rizvi, Fazal, and Bob Lingard. 2000. "Globalization and Education: Complexities and Contingencies." *Educational Theory* 50(4): 419–26.

Rodney, Walter. 1981. *How Europe Underdeveloped Africa*. Washington, DC: Howard University Press.

Rotarou, Elena. 2014. "Tourism in Zanzibar: Challenges for Pro-Poor Growth." *Caderno Virtual de Turismo* 14(3): 250–64.

Rousselot, Juliette. 2010. "Women in Nairobi: Too Scared to Pee." Human Rights Now blog. Amnesty International July 20. blog.amnestyusa.org/africa/women-in-nairobi-too-scared-to-pee.

SADC/SARDC and others. 2012. *Zambezi River Basin Atlas of the Changing Environment*. SADC, SARDC, ZAMCOM, GRID-Arendal, UNEP. Gabarone, Harare, and Arendal.

Sahu, Janmejay. 2012. "Corruption and Human Rights in Indian Context: An Overview." In V.N. Vishwanathan, ed. *Corruption and Human Rights*. New Delhi: Allied Publishers.

Sanya, B.N. 2012. *The Confluence of Colonialism and Patriarchy: An Analysis of Luo Women's Relationship to Agency.* Master's thesis, Simmons College. Retrieved from WorldCat (OCLC Number 870442340).

Sanya, B.N., and P.W. Odero. 2017. "Feminist Articulations, Social Literacies, and Ubiquitous Technology Use in Kenya." *Policy Futures in Education*. DOI: 10.1177/1478210317713074.

Seers, Dudley. 1969. "The Meaning of Development." *International Development Review* 11(4): 2–6.

Shoeman, Maxi. 2004. "Where Are the Women and How Are They Today? An Overview of the SADC Region." In *The Gender Perspective: Innovations in Economy, Organization, and Health within the Southern African Development Community (SADC)*, Ingelore Welpe, Britta Thege, and Shirley Henderson, eds. Pp. 10–33. New York: Peter Lang.

Smith, M.I., Tanya Yatsunenko, Mark J. Manary, Indi Trehan, Rajhab Mkakosya, Jiye Cheng, Andrew L. Kau, Stephen S. Rich, Patrick Concannon, Josyf C. Mychaleckyj, Jie Liu, Eric Houpt, Jia V. Li, Elaine Holmes, Jeremy Nicholson, Dan Knights, Luke K. Ursell, Rob Knight, and Jeffrey I. Gordon. 2013. "Gut Microbiomes of Malawian Twin Pairs Discordant for Kwashiorkor." *Science* 339: 548–54. DOI: 10.1126/science.1229000.

Soboyeja, Winston Wole. 2013. "Ceramic Water Filtration: From Science to Tech and Applications." Paper presented at the Safe Global Water Summit, Arusha, Tanzania, February 1.

Sorrenson, M.P.K. 1965. *Origins of European Settlement in Kenya*. Nairobi: Oxford University Press.

Spivak, Gayatri Chakravorty. 1999. *A Critique of Postcolonial Reason*. Cambridge: Harvard University Press.

Spivak, Gayatri Chakravorty. 2004. "Righting Wrongs." *The South Atlantic Quarterly* 103 (2/3): 523–81.

Steady, Filomina Chioma. 1985. {1981}. *The Black Woman Cross-Culturally*. Rochester, VT: Schenkman Books.

Sudbury, Julia. 1998. *'Other Kinds of Dreams': Black Women's Organizations and the Politics of Transformation*. London: Routledge.

Sudman, Seymour. 1976. *Applied Sampling*. New York: Academic Press.

Tanzania Central Statistical Office [CSO] and Institute for Resource Development/Macro Systems. 2010. *Tanzania Demographic and Health Survey 2010*. Calverton, MD: Tanzania CSO and ICF Macro.

Tanzania Central Statistical Office [CSO] and Institute for Resource Development/Macro Systems. 2016. *Tanzania Demographic and Health Survey 2016*. Calverton, MD: Tanzania CSO and ICF Macro.

Tanzania Development Vision 2025. www.tanzania.go.tz.

Taylor, B. 2009. "Addressing the Sustainability Crisis: Lessons from Research on Managing Rural Water Projects." *Water Aid Tanzania*. wateraidtz@wateraid.org.

Terborg-Penn, Rosalyn, and Andrea Benton Rushing. 1996. *Women in Africa and the African Diaspora: A Reader*. Washington, DC: Howard University Press.

The Constitution of Kenya, 2010. 2010. www.refworld.org/docid/4c8508822.html.

Thiong'o, Ngugi wa. 1986. *Decolonising the Mind: The Politics of Language in African Literature*. Nairobi: East African Publishers.

Tiwari, Sangam. 2013. "Logistical Factors in WaSH Implementation for the Vulerable Population: Suitability, Convenience and Patience." Paper presented at the Safe Global Water Summit, Arusha, Tanzania, February 1.

Tolofari, Sowaribi. 2005. "New Public Management and Education." *Policy Futures in Education*, 3(1): 75–89.

Tsinda, Aime, Pamela Abbott, and Jonathan Chenoweth. 2015. "Sanitation Markets in Urban Informal Settlements of East Africa." *Habitat International* 49: 21–29.

Tuck, Eve, and K. Wayne Yang. 2012. "Decolonization Is Not a Metaphor." *Decolonization: Indigeneity, Education and Society* 1(1): 1–40.

Tumwebaze, Innocent K., and Hans-Joachim Mosler. 2014. "Shared Toilet Users' Collective Cleaning and Determinant Factors in Kampala Slums, Uganda." *Bio Med Central (BMC) Public Health* 14: 1260. DOI: 10.1186/1471-2458-14-1260.

Turpie, Jane, Yonika M. Ngaga, and Francis Karanja. 2005. *Catchment Ecosystems and Downstream Water: The Value of Water Resources in the Pangani Basin, Tanzania*. Lao PDR. IUCN Water, Nature and Economics Technical Paper No. 7. IUCN, The World Conservation Union, Ecosystems and Livelihoods Group Asia.

Uganda Bureau of Statistics [UBOS] and Institute for Resource Development/Macro Systems. 2011. *Uganda Demographic and Health Survey 2011*. Kampala: UBOS and ICF International.

Ullman, Richard. 1978. "Human Rights and Economic Power: The United States Versus Idi Amin." *Foreign Affairs* (April 1978): 529–43. https://www.foreignaffairs.com/articles/uganda/1978-04-01/human-rights-and-economic-power-united-states-versus-idi-amin.

UNAIDS Country Factsheets Kenya http://www.unaids.org/en/regionscountries/countries/kenya

UNESCO and International Social Science Council. 2010. *World Social Science Reports, Knowledge Divides*. Paris: UNESCO and ISSC.

UNHCR. 1997. "Refugees in Western Tanzania: The Distribution of Burdens and Benefits Among Local Hosts." *Journal of Refugee Studies* 15: 339–58. DOI: 10.1093/jrs/15.4.339.

UNHCR. *UNHCR in 2016*. 2016a. New York: United Nations. www.unhcr.org/globaltrends2016.

UNHCR. 2016b. *Southern Sudan Regional Response Plan*. New York: United Nations.

UNHCR. 2017. *Global Focus–Uganda*. New York: United Nations. reporting.unhcr.org/node/5129.

UN-Habitat. 2009. *Tanzania: Dar es Salaam City Profile*. Nairobi: United Nations Human Settlements Programme.

UNICEF. 2003. *WASH and Women*. UNICEF. www.unicef.org/wash/index_womenandgirls.html.

UNICEF. 2016. *Gender and Water, Sanitation and Hygiene (WASH)*. UNICEF. https://www.unicef.org/esaro/7310_Gender_and_WASH.html.

United Nations. 2008. *Millennium Development Goals Report*. New York: United Nations.

United Nations. 2010. "Resolution adopted by the General Assembly, Sixty Fourth Session," agenda item 48. New York: United Nations.

United Nations. 2014. *The UN-Water Global Analysis and Assessment of Sanitation and Drinking-Water (GLAAS) Report: Investing in Water and Sanitation: Increasing Access, Reducing Inequalities*. World Health Organization: Geneva.

United Nations. 2015. *Transforming our World: The 2030 Agenda for Sustainable Development*. www.un.org/sustainabledevelopment/development-agenda.

United Nations. 2017. *Zero Hunger*. https://sr.one.un.org/2-zero-hunger.

United Nations Inter-Agency Group for Child Mortality Estimation (IGME). 2014. *Levels and Trends in Child Mortality, Report 2014*. www.un.org/en/development/desa/population/publications/mortality/child-mortality-report-2015; www.childmortality.org.

United Nations Office of the High Commissioner for Human Rights, United Nations Human Settlements Programme (UN-Habitat), and the World Health Organization. 2010. *The Right to Water*, Fact Sheet No. 35. www.ohchr.org/Documents/Publications/FactSheet35en.pdf.

United Republic of Tanzania. 1981. *The United Republic of Tanzania*. Water Utilization (Control and Regulation [Amendment]) Act. No. 10 of 1981, Tanzania. Dar es Salaam: Government Printer.

United Republic of Tanzania. 2002a. *National Water Policy. Ministry of Water and Livestock Development*. Dar es Salaam: Government Printer.

United Republic of Tanzania. 2002b. *National Strategy for Gender Development (NSGD). Ministry of Community Development, Gender and Children*. Dar es Salaam; Government Printer.

United Republic of Tanzania. 2005. *National Strategy for the Growth and Reduction of Poverty*. Vice President's Office Dar-es Salaam, Tanzania. http://www.povertymonitoring.go.tz.

United Republic of Tanzania. 2008. *National Water Sector Development Strategy. Ministry of Water and Irrigation 2006–2015*. Dar es salaam: Government Printer. *https://www.maji.go.tz/sites/default/files/u12/natinalwaterstrategy1.pdf.*

United Republic of Tanzania. 2009. *Water Resources Management Act No. 11*. Ministry of Water, United Republic of Tanzania. Dar es Salaam: Government Printer.

United Republic of Tanzania. 2010. *Ministry of Finance: Budget Speech on the Estimates of the Government Revenue and Expenditure for the Financial Year 2010/2011*. Dar es Salaam: Government Printer.

University of Illinois Board of Trustees. 2017. "Safe Global Water Institute: About Us." publish.illinois.edu/safeglobalwater/about-sgwi.

van Vliet, Bas J. van Buuren, P. Oosterveer, and G. Spaargaren. 2014. "Network Governance and Waste and Sanitation Service Provision: An Introduction to the Modernized Mixtures Approach." In *Urban Waste and Sanitation Services for Sustainable Development: Harnessing Social and Technical Diversity in East Africa, 9–96*. New York: Routledge.

Wanjala, Bernadette M., and Roldan Muradian. 2013. "Can Big Push Interventions Take Small-Scale Farmers Out of Poverty? Insights from the Sauri Millennium Village in Kenya." *World Development* 45: 147–60.

Waris, Attiya, Matti Kohonen, Jack Ranguma, and Alvin Mosioma. 2009. *Taxation and State Building in Kenya: Enhancing Revenue Capacity to Advance Human Welfare*. Nairobi: Tax Justice Network Africa.

Wasonga, Job, Mark Okowa, and Felix Kioli. 2016. "Sociocultural Determinants to Adoption of Safe Water, Sanitation and Hygiene Practices in Nyakach, Kisumu County, Kenya: A Descriptive Qualitative Study." *Journal of Anthropology*. DOI: 7434328.

Watanabe, K., and Petri, W.A. 2016. "Environmental Enteropathy: Elusive but Significant Subclinical Abnormalities in Developing Countries." *EBioMedicine* 10: 25–32. DOI: 10.1016/j.ebiom.2016.07.030.

Weintstein, Lena. 2008. "The New Scramble for Africa." *International Socialist* Review 60: July–August.

West, Michael O. 2002. *The Rise of an African Middle Class: Colonial Zimbabwe 1898–1965*. Bloomington and Indianapolis: University of Indiana Press.

West, Michael O. 2005. "Global Africa: The Emergence and Evolution of an Idea." *Review: A Journal of the Fernand Braudel Center* 28: 85–108.

West, Michael O. 2016. Personal communication.

Whitaker, Beth Elise. 2002. "Refugees in Western Tanzania: The Distribution of Burdens and Benefits among Local Hosts." *Journal of Refugee Studies* 15: 339–58. DOI: 10.1093/jrs/15.4.339.

White, Howard. 2002. "Combining Quantitative and Qualitative Approaches in Poverty Analysis." *World Development* 30(3): 511–22.

White, Linda B. 2014. "Hygiene Hypothesis: Why It May Be OK to Get a Little Dirty." *Mother Earth News*, November 26. https://www.motherearthnews.com/natural-health/hygiene-hypothesis-zm0z14djzsor.

Wilkinson, John Gardner. 1841. *A Second Series of the Manners and Customs of the Ancient Egyptians including Their Religion, Agriculture: Derived from a Comparison of the Paintings, Sculptures, and Monuments Still Existing, with the Accounts of Ancient Authors. Volume 1.* London: J. Murray.

WHO/UNICEF Joint Monitoring Programme for Water Supply and Sanitation. 2014. *Estimates on the Use of Water Sources and Sanitation.*

WHO/UNICEF Joint Monitoring Programme for Water Supply and Sanitation. 2015. *Estimates on the Use of Water Sources and Sanitation.* https://www.wssinfo.org/data-estimates.

Wolfe, P. 2006. "Settler Colonialism and the Elimination of the Native." *Journal of Genocide Research* 8(4): 387–409. DOI: 10.1080/14623520601056240.

World Bank. 2004. *River Basin Management and Smallholder Irrigation Improvement Project (RBMSIIP).* Implementation Completion report, Africa Region. Report No: 30929.

World Bank. 2011. *World Development Report—Gender Equality and Development.* International Bank for Reconstruction and Development/World Bank.

World Bank. 2012. *The World Development Report. Gender Equality and Development. The International Bank for Reconstruction and Development.* Washington DC: World Bank.

World Bank. 2013. *Global Monitoring Report 2013: Rural-Urban Dynamics and the Millennium Development Goals.* Washington DC: World Bank and the International Monetary Fund 2013 International Bank for Reconstruction and Development.

World Bank. 2015, March. *Uganda Economic Update,* 5th ed. *The Growth Challenge: Can Ugandan Cities Get to Work?* www.worldbank.org/en/country/uganda/brief/uganda-economic-update-fifth-edition-the-growth-challenge-can-ugandan-cities-get-to-work-fact-sheet.print.

World Bank. 2016a. "Poverty and Equity: Kenya." povertydata.worldbank.org/poverty/country/KEN.

World Bank. 2016b. "Poverty and Equity: Tanzania." povertydata.worldbank.org/poverty/country/TZA.

World Bank. 2016c. "Poverty and Equity: Uganda." povertydata.worldbank.org/poverty/country/UGA.

World Bank. 2016d. *World Bank East Asia and Pacific Economic Update April 2016: Growing Challenges. Washington DC: 2016 International Bank for Reconstruction and Development.*

World Health Organization. 2006. *Expanding Data Collection.* www.who.int/water_sanitation_health/monitoring/collection.pdf.

World Health Organization. 2014. *Investing in Water and Sanitation: Increasing Access, Reducing Inequalities.* UN Water Global Analysis and Assessment of Sanitation and Drinking Water (GLAAS). Geneva, Switzerland. https://www.wssinfo.org/documents/?tx_displaycontroller[type]=country_files.

Yamane, T. 1967. *Statistics: An Introductory Analysis*, 2nd ed. New York: Harper and Row.

Yuval-Davis, N., 1997. *Gender and Nation.* London: Sage Publications.

Zeleza, Paul Tiyambe. 1992. "The Colonial Labour System in Kenya." In *An Economic History of Kenya*, W.R. Ochieng and R.M. Maxon, eds. Pp. 171–200. Nairobi: East Africa Educational Publishers.

Zerai, Assata. 2014. *Hypermasculinity and State Violence in Zimbabwe Undermining Family Wellbeing: An African Feminist Analysis of Maternal and Child Health. Trenton, NJ:* Africa World Press.

Zerai, Assata, and Rae Banks. 2002. *Dehumanizing Discourse, Anti-Drug Law and Policy in America: A "Crack Mother's Nightmare."* Aldershot, England: Ashgate Publishing.

Zerai, Assata, T. Olemako, R. Morrow, and J. Guest. 2017. *An Interdisciplinary Analytical Framework to Understand Socioeconomic and Cultural Contexts for Delivery of Safe Water, Sanitation, and Resource Management in Refugee Settlements and Host Communities in Uganda*. Social and Behavioral Sciences Research Initiative (SBSRI) Small Grant Project Proposal. University of Illinois.

Zerai, Assata, Joanna Perez, and Chenyi Wang. 2016. "A Proposal for Expanding Endarkened Transnational Feminist Praxis: Creating a Database of Women's Scholarship and Activism to Promote Health in Zimbabwe." *Qualitative Inquiry*. DOI: 10.1177/1077800416660577.

Zinn, Maxine Baca, Lynn Weber Cannon, Elizabeth Higginbotham, and Bonnie Thornton Dill. 1986. "The Cost of Exclusionary Practices in Women's Studies." *Signs* 11: 290–303.

Index

About the Contributors

Assata Zerai, PhD, professor of sociology at the University of Illinois at Urbana Champaign since 2002, is a core affiliate faculty member in and former director of the Center for African Studies. She received her PhD in sociology from the University of Chicago. Zerai's research frameworks (theory and methodology) build from Black feminist thought, intersectionality, and African and African feminisms. Zerai's interests have included maternal and child health, health activism, safe water and sanitation, and ICTs (information and communications technologies) in Africa and the African diaspora as well as U.S.-based studies of women's health, diversity, and LGBTIQQ inclusiveness in Protestant congregations and making the work of indigenous and marginalized scholars and activists more accessible. Zerai's recent books include *Intersectionality in Intentional Communities: The Struggle for Inclusivity in Multicultural U.S. Protestant Congregations* (Rowman & Littlefield, Lexington Books, 2016) and *Hypermasculinity and State Violence in Zimbabwe: An African Feminist Analysis of Maternal and Child Health* (Africa World Press, 2014). She is author of *Dehumanizing Discourse, Law and Policy in America: A Crack Mother's Nightmare* (with Rae Banks, Ashgate 2002).

Brenda N. Sanya, PhD, is A. Lindsay O'Connor visiting assistant professor of educational studies at Colgate University. She received a PhD in global studies in education with a minor in queer studies at the University of Illinois at Urbana Champaign, where she was also a Cultures of Law in Global Contexts fellow. She received her MA in gender and cultural studies at Simmons College in Boston. Broadly, Sanya's research in Kenya and in the United States is animated by questions about how structural inequalities which marginalize people based on race, class, gender, and sexuality can erase or render precarious legal rights and privileges. To that end, her scholarship examines the limits of advantages provided by education, how education functions as a mediator for constitutional rights and citizenship and immigration rights for minoritized peoples, and the discretionary application of laws. Sanya's work has been published in *Feminist Africa, Gender and Education, Left History, Transnational Social Review, Policy Futures in Education*, and edited collections including *The Role of Civil Society in the Emancipation of Women, Mobilizing Identities*, and *Kenya after Fifty*. She is currently co-editing "Educative Practices and the Making of (Non)Citizens," a special issue for *Curriculum Inquiry* journal.

Teresia R. Olemako, PhD, is a research scientist in the Department of Geography and Geographic Information Science at the University of Illinois at Urbana Champaign. Olemako's current research project is entitled "Energy Access, Entrepreneurship and Women's Development in Urban Areas of Dar es Salaam, Tanzania" under her department's Social Dimensions of Environmental Policy. Olemako also works with NGOs and colleges in Tanzania to design online training for women and gender development studies. She served as a programme coordinator for extractives and renewable energy at the World Wildlife Fund (WWF) Tanzania country office. Her main role has been working with women, civil society organizations, and local communities to provide sustainable clean energy solutions. Olemako also contributes to shifting the world to a low-carbon economy by engaging with other stakeholders within the WWF global network and the government and private sectors. To achieve this end, she works hard to ensure increasing use of clean, renewable energy and promoting greater energy efficiency as outlined in the Sustainable Energy for All (SE4ALL) initiative by 2030. For approximately 18 years, she was a lecturer in the College of African Wildlife Management Mweka and a community conservation officer in Tanzania National Parks (TANAPA). A Tanzanian, Olemako has a PhD in development studies from Sokoine University of Agriculture, Tanzania; a master's degree in community economic development from Southern New Hampshire University; and a postgraduate diploma in wildlife management from the College of African Wildlife Management Mweka, Tanzania.

Rebecca L. Morrow, MA and a doctoral candidate in the Department of Sociology at the University of Illinois at Urbana Champaign, is completing her dissertation, *"That's Why We Always Fight Back": A Decolonized Feminist Life Course Analyzing Resistance and Resiliency Strategies of Native American Women*. Morrow received an MA in sociology from Western Illinois University in 2010. She has manuscripts under review by *Social Science and Medicine* and the *African Journal of Reproductive Health*. She is a part of the Safe Global Water Network, which seeks to provide sustainable, safe water and sanitation solutions while considering cultural contexts, especially gender. Morrow teaches a course in criminology and has served as a teaching assistant for Africa in the Global Perspective; Intro to Sociology; and Criminology, Deviance, and the Criminal Justice System. She uses an intersectional framework to study health, specifically children's health, reproductive health, and intimate partner violence in societies with severe structural violence, including countries of the Global South, Native American reservations, and prisons.

Courtney Cuthbertson, PhD, is an evaluation and community behavioral health specialist in Extension at Michigan State University. She earned her PhD in sociology from the University of Illinois at Urbana Champaign in 2014 and served as a postdoctoral fellow in community behavioral health for the North Central Regional Center for Rural Development. Her research examines the social and biomedical processes through which impactful or traumatic social events are recast as issues of individual illness and pathology. Cuthbertson's dissertation investigated how global mental health knowledge shaped lived experiences of depression in Chile; biomedicine was perceived by interviewees not to resolve issues creating distress but to enable them to withstand unchangeable social circumstances. Cuthbertson has also investigated mental health consequences of the Flint water crisis, finding that community leaders perceive lack of government responsiveness to residents' claims of health problems as potentially more impactful on mental health than the uncertainty of whether one would experience physical health consequences from consuming lead-contaminated water. Her work has been published in *Journal of Urban Health*, *Journal of Affective Disorders*, and *Transgressive Culture*.

Joanna B. Perez, PhD, is an assistant professor of sociology at California State University, Dominguez Hills. She received her BA in sociology from UCLA, with a double minor in labor and workplace studies and civic engagement. More recently, Perez received an MA and a PhD in sociology with a minor in Latina/Latino Studies from the University of Illinois at Urbana Champaign. She is a recipient of the American Sociological Association (ASA) Minority Fellowship and the Fund for the Advancement of the Discipline (FAD) grant. Since starting her postsecondary education trajectory as a scholar activist, her research has explored the ways that marginalized communities challenge systems of power and social inequality through activism in order to alter their social position and advocate for social change. In particular, she is working on a book manuscript that contextualizes the experiences of Latina/o undocumented immigrant young adult activists in the U.S. Her recent co-authored publications include: *"Ni de aqui, ni de alla": Undocumented Immigrant Youth and the Challenges of Identity Formation amid Conflicting Contexts* and *A Proposal for Expanding Endarkened Transnational Feminist Praxis: Creating a Database of Women's Scholarship and Activism to Promote Health in Zimbabwe*. Her areas of specialization include Latina/o sociology; immigration; family; racial and ethnic minorities; law and society; social movements; and qualitative methodology.

Shorma Bianca Bailey, MS, is a doctoral student in the Department of Agricultural and Biological Engineering at the University of Illinois at Urbana Champaign. Her dissertation focuses on the investigation of an onsite agricultural water treatment system for developing and developed worlds. Formerly she was president of the Howard University Chapter of Engineers without Borders. She completed installing water filters in a rural village in Kenya, benefiting members of the Kenyan community, who gained access to clean water. Bailey's other international research was conducted in Sudan, Nepal, and most recently South Africa.

As a result of her international work, in 2011 Bianca was named a White House Champion of Change for women and girls in science and engineering. She has worked in chemical engineering, environmental engineering, nanotechnology, and agriculture. She looks forward to graduation and starting her career in international development.

www.ingramcontent.com/pod-product-compliance
Lightning Source LLC
Chambersburg PA
CBHW051252200926
51612CB00001B/14
9781498520836